THE SECRET OF STAYING YOUNG

Age Reversal for Mind & Body

DR. MARIE MICZAK

LOTUS

DISCLAIMER

This book is not a substitute for professional medical care and should be utilized with common sense and under the advice of your health care professional. The author and publisher are therefore not responsible for use of the information in this book used outside of the scope for which it is intended, that being under your physician's supervision.

COVER & PAGE DESIGN/LAYOUT: Paul Bond, Art & Soul Design

First Edition, 2001

Printed in the United States of America

The Secret of Staying Young: Age Reversal for Mind & Body
ISBN 0-910261-33-4
Library of Congress Control Number: 2001132216

Published by:
Lotus Press, P.O. Box 325, Twin Lakes, Wisconsin 53181
web: www.lotuspress.com
e-mail: lotuspress@lotuspress.com
800-824-6396

TABLE OF CONTENTS

■

DEDICATION

■

This book is dedicated to
my beautiful Gina Magda, (the Hungarian Princess),
whose youthful curiosity, humor
and wit inspires me each day.
I love you so very much.

INTRODUCTION

∎

Today there is an ever-expanding amount of choices for consumers. An emerging branch of food supplements, called nutricueticals, have made their presence felt in both the media and in the market. Nutriceuticals is a term used to describe nutrients that are demonstrating medicinal qualities. Examples would be Gingko Biloba, which in and among other things helps increase blood flow to the brain. Sales of this category of herbal and nutritional supplements has more than doubled in the past 4 years in the United States alone. The average consumer, however, usually does not have enough information to determine which products are really helpful and which are only hype. Adding to the problem of the public's quest for information is the Internet. Many people hope to read about a nutritional supplement online as a way of gathering information. The problem is that many websites are owned by vitamin or herb companies. Therefore the information they present may be biased in favor of the benefits as opposed to discussing the risks of their products.

Since herbs and food supplements are a property of public domain, most pharmaceutical companies prefer to put their research dollar into developing synthetic or laboratory created drugs, not herbs. This is due to the fact that drug companies will spend upwards of 800 million dollars to bring a new drug to market. Herbal and nutritional supplements being unpatentable means that the drug manufactures would never regain their research and development costs. Even taking this point into consideration, we owe up to 40% of the medications being prescribed today to plants and natural compounds. There is also little thought given to the fact that many of these natural products have a longer track record for both usefulness and safety than many newer prescriptions.

Right now as the population of "baby boomers" ages, nutriceuticals that may assist in addressing the maladies associated with the aging process are highly desirable. This is because the population over age 65 is increasing. Right now in America, this age group is 10 million strong. By the year 2030 we can expect this group to double to 20 million. What does this mean? Well, we are going to see more elderly people taking care of their parents in their advanced years. For example, once you reach 65, you will most likely be caring for one or more aged parents or in-laws in their late eighties to nineties.

We are actually beginning to see this trend now. In order to add support to the limits of Social Security, President Clinton has signed a bill that will allow older Americans to work while collecting their check. This is in part out of necessity because when Social Security was first instituted during the Delanor Roosevelt administration, the life expectancy of the average American was much lower. Therefore the amount of money taken out of wages would carry a person about 5-8 years after retirement. This is far too little for people who are now living 10, 20 or 30 years after collecting their last pay check.

Such changes have sent shock waves through the government's ability to guarantee that Social Security will still be there. The fact is, this money has been in trouble for years. This is because most Americans who have been collecting Social Security for more than ten years have more than gotten double what they actually paid into it. So it is the money from current wage earners that is going into this retirement fund, paying current recipients and not being set aside for future ones.

With Social Security on the verge of collapse, you will see people having to work longer. They will also have to be quite savvy about managing their retirement packages as well. Whatever must be done, will you be up to the task? What about the quality of your life? Longevity is not much to speak of if you are simply vegetating in a nursing home. I think we all expect that we will be fully functioning mentally and physically until our last breath. The reality of the matter is much grimmer. Another point is that even if you have some measure of health, but not enough money to support yourself, many families will admit such ones into a nursing home. You do not have enough money to be the master of your destiny any longer, so someone else makes this decision for you. Will you be happy with that?

While there is no magic bullet and consumers should not be expected to take an herb or any other food supplement on blind faith, there is fascinating new information being released as to the benefits of such on the human system. I believe that where such evidence exists as to the positive effects of an herb or supplement, that no entity has the power to restrict public access to this information in the interest of private industry and their lobbyists. Much of what we are allowed to use as far as medicines is directly related to this fact.

By actually addressing the underlying causes of many illnesses and conditions related to aging, we can identify substances that may be both safe and effective in combating them. Traditionally, in medicine today the elderly are treated with sympathy, but not the aggressive conviction reserved for younger patients. Older patients are often patted on the hand and told, "Well, you know you are getting up in age and this problem is quite common among the elderly." This is cold comfort for someone who came to his or her doctor for help, not terms of surrender. We all want to be respected as individuals even in our senior years. A condescending pat on the back is not what health consumers are paying for, young or old.

For example, chemical imbalance in the brain is often seen to be at the root of many mental disorders such as compulsive-obsessive and depression. Accepted medical practice advocates their correction, which has shown documented relief of these problems. However, if we simply assume that all elderly patients eventually become depressed, will we then say that this is a part of getting old and not seek treatment for them? Another possibility, which I have seen in my own practice, is the routine administration of antidepressants to elderly patients without any real evaluation of whether they are depressed or not. Zoloft, (sertraline), is often the drug of choice for this age group and may most often be prescribed by the patient's general practitioner without a proper psychological check up.

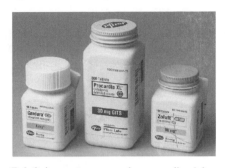

Zoloft is most commonly prescribed for elder depression but interacts with medications older patients may already be on such as Procardia XL. Zoloft taken with nifedipine can cause toxicity.

So this is what we are up against. The time to prepare yourself is now. It is never too late to improve the quality of your life at any age, but of course to get the most benefit, you will want to start as soon as possible. First look at these statistics:

• In 1996 the oldest of the Baby Boomers born between 1946 and 1964, turned 50.

• In 1996 Baby Boomers represented close to 30% of the population in America.

• People aged 50+ have an average income of $44,000 with over 10 percent of that amount being discretionary income.

• Only 1 in 3 retirees has a pension

• 95 million Americans have little or no health insurance

This book will give you a philosophy that you can apply to take control of your health. You will also learn what wonderful nutritional products you can and should add to your daily program to help you look and feel your best. Maintaining peak mental performance and memory retention is also at issue as we age, as well as the growing frequency of Alzheimer's disease. Osteoporosis and cardiac disease will also be thoroughly discussed with ideas, nutrients, herbs and foods recommended for each. Lastly, skin and body care products you can make at home to improve your skin's health and youthful appearance is covered. A total rejuvenation package!

Chapter 1

YOUR PERSONAL EVALUATION

■

One of the main dilemmas in health care research today is quality of life vs. quantity of years. The technology is now available to keep a patient alive even without the spontaneous reflex of breathing or physically feeding oneself. For example, many Americans are living in nursing homes while given a minimally nutritious diet and exercise.

Although most often such institutions meal plans are under the guidance of a registered dietitian, it is estimated that close to 40% of patients admitted into hospitals leave suffering from malnutrition even though they entered relatively well nourished. It would not be fair to entirely blame the dietitians in charge of the food service at such institutions, but the system that allows them to choose the foods served most certainly contributes to it. This is because dietitians are concerned with feeding large populations of institutionalized patients for a certain dollar amount. In fact many dietitians were trained under the Home Economics departments of their schools or colleges. So nutrition is of some importance, but feeding still takes precedence.

Often times people look to physicians for a cure yet over-look other lifestyle factors that can add health and longevity to their benefit. Not recognizing your own need for personal choice and empowerment when making health care decisions

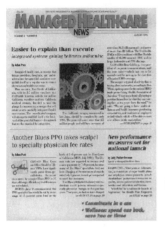 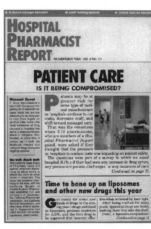 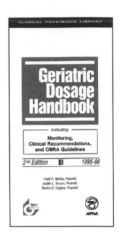

Above Left, This is a trade magazine for health care cost managers designed to keep an eye on the bottom line; Above Center, Geared to the specific needs of hospital pharmacists who are restricted to the use of certain drugs chosen by the hospital administrators, many of whom are not medical professionals; Above Right, This handbook addresses the specific needs of elderly patients for drug absorption and excretion.

shows the practitioner that you have not put a vested interest into getting better. This lack of taking responsibility is likely at the root of the medical profession's "giving up" on someone who in their opinion has reached the end of his or her useful-ness. In other words, unless you get interested and start ask-ing questions, your doctor may just give you something to treat the symptoms and not address the underlying causes of the condition. These underlying causes often start with poor lifestyle choices. Yes, we all know about smoking and exces-sive alcohol intake, but what about other things? What I mean are those hidden hydrogenated fats in our processed baked goods, lead in our water, pesticide residue on our fruits and vegetables. This list expands. Now before you give up and say,

"Well then everything is poison, I guess." consider that life can and does go on and that there are a handful of individuals who have mastered the secrets to avoid many of these issues, thus improving their health into their advancing years.

Starting with yourself, consider how one's attitudes, beliefs and prejudices all play into the support of the status quo in the treatment of older patients. If we can be objective and honest at the same time, what are our own true feelings when we are stuck behind a senior citizen in traffic? Do we think that they are too old to drive, an accident waiting to happen? Do we feel that they should simply get off the road, pack it in and stay home? If so, we have to realize that this is a conditioned response. Even insurance companies know that newly licensed drivers account for most of the motor vehicle accidents and charge them accordingly on their premiums. We are encouraged to believe that as we age, we must accept any and all decline in mental ability, memory and speed of reflex, no matter what the underlying cause. By shutting the door on looking into what may be causing the problem, we also close the door on discovering their respective solution.

Statistics on Aging:

* Average life expectancy for an American male as of 1984 is 71.5 years whereas women can expect to live 78.2 years. (This gap is ever narrowing due to the increase of women smokers over the years.)
* Senior citizens actually call out sick less than their younger worker counterparts.
* Only one out of every three retired workers has a pension.

Behind these numbers is the fact that most seniors live on a fixed income. Food and utility prices rise quarterly while cost of living increases for pensions and Social Security often lag sorely behind. Attitudes of the elderly about what their bodies actually need likewise keep them from spending any extra money on high quality foods and dietary supplements. This is because many grew up during the great depression and saw their families make do with white bread, potatoes and hot dogs. The fact that they survived to their advanced age may make them think that good nutrition is not really that important but a full stomach is. So foods may be chosen for cost-effectiveness, not quality.

If the elderly can look beyond these deeply entrenched responses, they will see that they can do much to improve the quality of their lives just like other members of society. I was employed in a pharmacy that served nursing homes several years ago. Some did receive a daily dose of synthetic liquid vitamins, (coal tar derivatives), but by far most were over-medicated with depressants and sedatives. Prime candidates for this sort of numbing therapy include patients who may demand too much attention than the nursing home staff can provide. Cut-backs equal perhaps only a few qualified nurses on the floor, with the bulk of the nursing staff consisting of nurse's aids, who do not have the same level of training to deal with patient care. Therefore it is not difficult to see how many nursing home residents become labeled "problem patients".

Due to these stereotypes, many also accept all the ailments of the elderly as part of the natural life cycle of man. Less effort may be put into treating the elderly even though many of their health problems are not age related. In many cultures, putting the aged outside the village to die or be eaten by wild animals was a way to deal with a person who has outlived his usefulness and is now just consuming scarce resources. This survivalist mentality is still alive and well in even the most "civilized" societies such as our own. Deep inside are we too quick to accept the premature passage of our elders? Could this be due to pressures on food supplies as the world's population continues to soar along with hunger and third world poverty?

Even with these conditioned responses, it must be noted that many of the physical effects of aging can be addressed and often reversed. Case in point; if a young person develops cataracts, eye surgery is quickly scheduled to restore normal vision. When an elderly patient presents the same condition, doctors may simply chalk it up to old age and perhaps not even recommend operating. This is often true if the person is being cared for and not living independently. The technology and procedure is exactly the same for cataract removal for both age groups. Yet the view of the older patient's needs and value as a human being are quite different from his or her younger counterpart.

"She has her whole life ahead of her." "He has so much to live for." These thoughts are often not expressed in describing older people. However, in reality for any one of us a whole life ahead could mean 30 years or even 30 minutes. The Bible poetically calls our attention to the fact that tomorrow is not promised to us. No one is assured to live the next day or the next minute for that matter. Youth is therefore no absolute guarantee of longevity, either.

Chapter 2

SUGGESTED SUPPLEMENTATION FOR OLDER ADULTS
(Who Want to Feel Younger!)

■

This chapter will help you to develop a nutritional protocol designed to fit your specific needs. No matter where you are in age, there is much that you can and must do to feel and look your best. We are starting with the basics here but you will quickly see how other nutritional supplements or nutriceuticals can be used to offset many of the symptoms associated with aging. Actually much of what we assume is just part of getting old may be due to dietary deficiencies. These deficiencies are often made worse by the fact that as we get older, we may not be able to absorb the vitamins and minerals so easily assimilated in youth. Under each section of recommended minerals, vitamins and herbs, you will find informative articles on the why and how of each supplement as well as what it can do for you. The precise amounts of nutrients may vary depending on your age, weight and sex. That is why it is best to seek the guidance of a nutritionist or certified nutritional consultant. They will take into account any pre-existing medical conditions and problems that might make some supplements out of your reach.

Therefore, please view the following as basic guidelines upon which you can build the framework of your own personalized approach to health and longevity.

YOUR GENERAL GUIDE TO TAKING VITAMINS

Vitamins and minerals often interact with each other and with many foods. In some cases, these interactions boost absorption. In others, they block it. Some guidelines to make sure you are getting, and absorbing, what you need:

- Do not down handfuls of pills at a time. Our ability to absorb megadoses or multidoses is limited and the excess will only be excreted in the urine. Try taking small amounts throughout the day with meals as most vitamins will "piggyback" on a protein molecule therefore being absorbed more readily.

- Avoid taking calcium at the same meal with multivitamins or with supplements containing either iron or zinc. Calcium blocks their absorption. Instead, take your calcium at night, away from other supplements and medicines when it will have a better chance of being absorbed into your bones.

- Vitamin C boosts the absorption of iron. Taking a supplement with both vitamin C and iron together increases the bioavailability and assimilation of the iron.

- Iron and calcium are both better tolerated with food, although their absorption is slightly decreased. Fat-soluble vitamins - A, D, E and K - are better absorbed with food, especially meals containing some fat.

Keep in mind that mineral supplements such as calcium may have naturally occurring heavy metal contaminants. An example being calcium supplements, which are originally derived from ground limestone, (calcium carbonate), bonemeal or oyster shells. They could easily have higher than allowed concentrations of lead. To add insult to injury, most of the limestone and oyster shell products are not very bioavailable and therefore will do your bones little or no good while collecting in your soft tissues! This is how kidney stones are born.

ARE YOU BONING UP ON CALCIUM?
"The Best Type of Calcium for You and Your Bones"

Today there are a variety of vitamin supplements on the market. Calcium carbonates found in inexpensive products such as Caltrate may not be adequately absorbed. Women need between 1,000 - 1,500 mgs of elemental calcium daily to insure not only optimal bone density but proper heart and neurological function as well.

Additionally, our bodies can only absorb up to 600 mgs of calcium at a time so megadosing may do more harm than good. Also timing is essential. Taking calcium before bedtime could help insure that it gets into the bones and is not used up by competing muscle cells trying to displace lactic acid.

Dietary sources are a good place to start, but do not put too much stock in dairy products. Scandinavians are the world's largest consumers of milk products, yet have the highest incidence of osteoporosis. Broccoli, collard greens, sesame seeds and sardines with bones are all appreciably high in calcium.

Traditionally, Native American Indian women have used Rubus idaeus, or red raspberry leaves, as an absorbable source of both calcium and its helper, magnesium, along with other trace minerals that are naturally balanced. They also ate fish liver, which is rich in preformed vitamin A and vitamin D. All of these provided a synergistic approach to building and maintaining bone density well into old age. (For more information see The Medicine Pouch chapter of *Nature's Weeds, Native Medicine...Native American Herbal Secrets*, Lotus Press)

Today, especially, it may be difficult to get the right amount of calcium from your diet. Other factors such as low hydrochloric acid in the stomach and aversion or allergies to many calcium rich foods may make matters worse. Calcium supplements of choice today include calcium citrates and a new substance called microcrystalline hydroxyapatite, the only form of calcium being reviewed by the FDA for the actual reversal of osteoporosis.

The best advice perhaps might be to take a cue from my Native American ancestors. The combination of diet, exercise, sun and herbs provided a multidirectional approach for a people who had no knowledge or tolerance for milk products or calcium supplements.

MAGNESIUM'S LINK TO HEART HEALTH
"Its Role in Fighting Heart Disease"

While scientists have long known that heart disease is less common in areas where drinking water naturally contains a lot of dissolved magnesium and other mineral salts, they have not known until recently to what extent a dietary deficiency of magnesium could effect human health.

Now Swiss researchers have found that people diagnosed with coronary heart disease have lower than normal levels of magnesium in their red blood cells. After six months of taking a magnesium supplement, researchers found that the attacks of severe chest pain were significantly decreased. Another key piece to this puzzle is the fact that the aspirin used in American studies linking it to a decrease in subsequent heart attacks was buffered. The buffering agent used in this type of aspirin is, you guessed it, magnesium!

Nutrition experts guess that about 90% of all Americans are at risk of magnesium deficiencies. The best dietary sources are dark, leafy green vegetables such as kale, turnip and collard greens to name a few.

Recommended magnesium supplementation stands at 50 mgs each of both magnesium orotate and magnesium aspartate. Chelated mineral supplements are also somewhat better absorbed than non-chelated.

Minerals such as calcium and magnesium are needed to

avoid more than just the ravages of osteoporosis. They also play an important role in heart and muscle function. The trace mineral Selenium has been thought to help prevent many kinds of cancer. Incidence of cancer increases with age so this is one trace mineral everyone should take. According to the *Journal of Practitioner's Health Alliance for Responsible Medicine* many studies have shown a correlation between fatal cancers and a selenium deficiency. Here is a reprint of that article under the Pharmacognosy column entitled:

THE SELENIUM SOLUTION
"May be Key to Preventing Many Cancers"

Although over consumption of selenium has in the past been suspect in the activation of some cancers, recent research has failed to substantiate earlier claims that selenium is carcinogenic, (cancer causing). Recently the tables have turned to in fact point to selenium as one of the most powerful cancer preventatives, (other than dietary and lifestyle changes), under investigation today. It might be interesting to note that as early as 1977, research was done into the relationship between low selenium intake and increased cancers. Age adjusted cancer mortalities were correlated with estimated selenium intakes in the U.S. and other nations calculated from food consumption data or by the actual measurement of selenium content of pooled blood. Significant inverse correlations were seen in cancers of the colon, rectum, prostate, breast, ovary and for leukemia. (Schrauzer GN et al. *Cancer mortality correlation studies-III: Statistical associations with dietary selenium intakes.* Bioorganic Chem. 7:23, 1977)

In 1985 results of a four-year study reported the following: 51 cancer patients involved in a case-controlled study investigated the relationship between serum concentrations of selenium as well as vitamins A and E. Fatal cancers corresponded to selenium deficiency. Vitamin E contributed to this effect and male smokers with both low selenium and low beta-carotene intake showed an increased incidence of lung cancer. *(Brit Med. J. 290:417, 1985)*

Selenium, as are vitamins A and E, is classified as an antioxidant, but unlike the latter two, selenium offers unique protection against cancer. In an observational study of 4,480 adults, the subsequent risk of developing cancer appears to be predicted by the serum selenium level, but not by the vitamin A carotenoid or vitamin E level. *(Nutr. Rev. 42(6):214-5, 1985)*

Just how much of this trace mineral do we need? Well it has been estimated that 250-300 mcgs. daily can prevent most cancers. In contrast the typical selenium consumption in the U.S. is only about 100 mcgs per day or only one-third of the amount recommended for cancer prevention. *(Schrazer, Gerhard, Ph.D. - 1981)*

BPH AND THE CADMIUM CONNECTION
"Zinc and Selenium May be the Solution"

Benign Prostatic Hyperplasia, or BPH, has long been considered a wake up call, (often in the middle of the night), to the male physiological changes to be anticipated in mid-life. After about age 50, a man's testosterone decreases while other hormones such as prolactin and estradiol increase. Enlargement of the prostate occurs when testosterone entering the prostate cell is converted to dihydrotestosterone. It is this substance, DHT, which enters the cell nucleus and stimulates protein synthesis, which then causes the abnormal growth and enlargement of the prostate. The prostate will progressively crowd the urethra that passes through it. The effect is much like someone standing on a garden hose, thus impeding the flow of water.

Damage to the kidneys and bladder infections are not uncommon with this condition. Primary symptoms include frequent trips to the bathroom and decreased urinary flow, which is evident in up to about 50% of all males by age sixty and close to 80% past age seventy. A total of close to 10 million American men are effected by this condition. Until recently, this was thought to be an inevitable part of the aging process. Now science has become aware of environmental and nutritional factors as playing a role in either helping or hindering this problem.

A controlled study showed that 14 out of 19 men exhibited improvement when they took the mineral zinc in the amount of 150 mgs daily for 2 months, with a maintenance dose of 50-100 mgs daily. This was demonstrated in 14 of the patients showing shrinkage of the prostate as assessed by rectal palpitation, X-ray and endoscopy. *(Bush IM et al Zinc and the Prostate)* Zinc is an essential mineral that is crucial to prostate gland function and the normal growth of reproductive organs. Deficiencies in zinc show up as hair loss, high cholesterol levels, impaired night vision, impotence, memory impairment and of course prostate trouble. The saddest part is all of these symptoms are associated with just getting older!

Not to be overlooked are our modern day exposures to chemicals and heavy metals, many of which are carcinogenic or cancer causing. One observational study took a close look at cadmium exposure. Cadmium is a soft bluish-white metal used industrially is electroplating, batteries and atomic reactors. Prostatic cadmium concentrations in patients with BPH were measured by atomic absorption spectroscopy and were found to be considerably higher than in normal tissue, (23.11 +/- 3.28 vs. 5.25 = /- 0.62 nmol/g). Prostatic DHT levels were directly proportional to the cadmium concentrations.

There seems to be evidence that selenium, mentioned previously for cancer prevention, may protect cadmium-induced growth stimulation of the prostatic tissue or epithelium. Patients may undertake a non-invasive elemental analysis that can assess both toxic cadmium and beneficial selenium / zinc ratios. This is accomplished through a simple hair analysis.

Suggested Daily Minerals:

1000-1,500 mgs of Calcium, (Preferably Cal-Apatite or Calcium Citrate)

200 mgs of Magnesium, (Chelated)

300 mcgs (note micrograms) of Selenium, a trace mineral

50-100 mgs of Zinc, (Chelated)

NOTE: *Many people opt for a complete multi-mineral supplement. This is fine but beware of high dosages of minerals as they can tax the kidneys and lead to their damage. If you purchase a multi- mineral product, make sure you have at least the amounts of those recommended above and not more.*

YOU ARE WHAT YOU ABSORB
"Why You May Need Digestive Enzymes"

It is a known fact that limiting the variety of foods consumed can cause a decrease in digestive enzymes. In my private practice as a certified nutritional consultant, I have seen many such cases over the years that prove this.

A forty-year-old woman came in complaining of gas and severe indigestion after eating practically anything. Her history as a recovering anorexic showed that she severely limited her food choices to about three items, crackers, cheese and peanut butter. After a while, any other food when introduced resulted in severe flatulence and dyspepsia.

She was given an array of digestive enzymes that would allow her to digest foods she had been avoiding such as meats, whole grains, vegetables and fruits. This allowed her to get some nourishment until her body could begin to produce more digestive enzymes. The theory as to why this happened is seen within the model of the problem many adults have with intolerance to lactose. Many of us drank milk as children but when we became adults we may have stopped. Therefore our bodies no longer produce lactase, which works on the substrate lactose. Here we can see that the body does not produce that which it does not need or use. In similar fashion, when we cut out entire food groups for long periods of time, you can't expect to instantly produce the enzymes to digest them when they are once again reintroduced. The more variety of foods this patient consumed, the more diverse enzymes she produced to digest them.

This patient was young and healthy. What about an older person? Well, special conditions apply here. Like this younger patient, older people begin restricting the variety of food they eat. Why? They are more likely to be on restricted diets due to high blood pressure, high cholesterol or adult on-set diabetes. Often times living on a fixed income, many seniors will buy the same foods for price value and ease of preparation. Other physiological factors also exist. For instance, as we get older we do not produce as much hydrochloric acid as we once did. This decrease can account for our inability to break down minerals such as calcium in our food and supplements. Taking products such as Tums to neutralize stomach acid only makes matters worse. In fact, a stomach that does not produce enough hydrochloric acid tends to churn *more* just to accomplish the initial breakdown of food. Therefore heartburn may be a sign that your stomach is producing too *little* acid.

Take a look at a child. How they can eat and with what crazy combinations! Yet, you seldom hear them complain of heartburn, gas or indigestion even after consuming large quantities of soda, cake and candy. This is because youth has endowed them with optimal amounts of both digestive enzymes and hydrochloric acid.

Recommended Digestive Enzymes:

Chewable Papaya with Enzymes, Papain, Lipase, Protease, etc. and HCL if needed

Take the chewable papaya before meals. People with ulcers

should not use any digestive enzyme formula with hydrochloric acid or HCL. Hydrochloric acid containing products should be taken *after* eating your meal for best results.

YOUR DAILY VITAMINS
"What and How Much to Take"

Nothing is more confusing than walking into a healthfood or drug store and being overwhelmed by the amount and variety of nutritional supplements available today. It is no coincidence either. Sales of nutritional supplements in the U.S. have showed steady gains over the years. For the first time you see mega pharmaceutical companies such as Merck and Johnson and Johnson's stocks drop. People have more access to reliable information, (such as the book you are now reading), and are willing to take more responsibility for their health.

During the 1970's, mega-dosing of vitamins was popular. This is when up to a thousand times more of the daily requirement for a nutrient was taken. The theory behind this method was to over-saturate the tissues and overcome deficiencies as quickly as possible. Certain vitamins are poorly absorbed from the stomach such as B-12. So injections of certain vitamins became popular because one could reach optimal serum levels in a few seconds, not days. Blood tests for vitamin deficiencies were also done. However, it was determined that this did not give an accurate indication of the level of that vitamin in the body. This is because blood tests only evaluate the amount of that nutrient circulating in the blood at that time. Vitamin levels will naturally be highest after a meal or taking a supplement.

Of particular concern is taking too much of fat-soluble vitamins, such as A and D, for example. Recent studies have shown excess vitamin A, (retinol) may be toxic and even increase the risk of birth defects. Therefore it is recommended that pregnant women and women of child bearing age take no more than 5,000 IU total of pre-formed vitamin A. Pre-formed vitamin A or retinol is found in fish liver oils such as cod and shark liver oil. It is called this because the vitamin A is pre-formed or manufactured in the fish's liver. It can cause liver damage if taken in high amounts. Beta-carotene, which is found in yellow and leafy green vegetables, is a different story. This form of vitamin A is converted only as needed by the liver, thus has little risk of toxicity from over-consumption.

Over time, processes such as chelation, (binding to a protein molecule), were developed in an effort to ensure better absorption of the nutrients in pill form. This is a major issue that will influence your purchasing choices of supplements. I teach a course called The Natural Pharmacy at Brookdale College in Lincroft, NJ where I have been adjunct faculty for more than 11 years. One of the things I show my students in this course is how vitamins will vary from brand to brand in your ability to absorb them.

To test to see how your vitamin stacks up, try this old method form my pharmaceutical research lab days. You will need the following equipment for this simple experiment:

Bioavailability Test

8 oz. of room temperature white vinegar

1 - 8 oz glass or beaker

Your favorite vitamin pill

Place your vitamin in the beaker of vinegar and let stand for 20-30 minutes at room temperature. Check the results after that time. Is the pill broken down into clumps or aggregates? If so this vitamin is most likely going to do the same when it meets your small intestine when digestion takes place. Is your pill still in one solid piece? Bad news then because that pill is just being passed through your digestive track without being broken down or absorbed!

So what can you do? Well, there are many options available today. One is to change your vitamin form. There are many vitamins available as chewable and liquid. One that I personally like is Floradix. This is a liquid vitamin supplement that is very easy to absorb. Another choice is adult chewables. Usually associated with children's vitamins, adult chewables offer an alternative to those who may have trouble swallowing large pills. When the vitamin is chewed it is broken down into the smaller, more absorbable aggregates previously mentioned. Not only that but there are natural enzymes present in your saliva that begin the digestion process right in your mouth. The result is getting everything you are supposed to out of that supplement.

Vitamin C has gotten so much attention over the last 20 years. Linus Pauling, the scientist who helped discover the structure of DNA, used it in high amounts and did many studies concerning its usefulness in combating disease. In fact, Pauling was a forerunner of a branch of medical science called orthomolecular medicine. Quite simply orthomolecular medicine deals with correcting deficiencies at the cellular level to promote normal function to the associated organs.

Pauling was ahead of his time as we are seeing vitamin deficiencies as being responsible for a whole host of symptoms once categorized as age related disorders.

Vitamin C should be taken in its buffered form. This is because high doses, or the cheaper and more common ascorbic acid, can cause excessive acidity in the body that can be harmful to delicate tissues. Healthy pH for the body is about 6.0 - 6.5. On the pH scale that runs from 1 to 14, a pH of 6.5 is just below neutral but a little on the acid side. This slight lean towards acidity helps protect the body from infection. Bacteria, yeasts and molds find an acidic pH to be a hostile environment for growth. Thus women especially with a urinary pH of 7 or higher, (alkaline), may find themselves much more susceptible to urinary tract infections. This is why cranberry juice and concentrates are often recommended for UTI's. The cranberry acidifies the urine and makes a hostile environment for the growth of germs.

Vitamin E or the d-alpha tocapherol (umbiquolone) should be a part of most everyone's vitamin repertoire. However, most clinical studies done involving vitamin E and heart health have used the natural of d-alpha tocapherol. This form seems to be more bioactive than the synthetic form. So when purchasing vitamin E capsules, you might wish to spend just a bit more to get the natural form. Like co-enzyme Q-10, vitamin E is very similar in molecular structure. It is likewise a very helpful antioxidant. People are able to see the benefits in short order, but beware as initial use of vitamin E can cause a temporary increase in blood pressure. You should acclimatize your system to its introduction by taking only 100 IU's per day for a week, adding 100 more IU's each week. This way you are slowly working up to 400 IU's over time.

B-complex vitamins should be taken just as that, in a complex. You will want to get all of the natural balance of the full array of B's, (B-1, B-2, B-6, etc.). This is because if you take more of just one of the B-complex vitamins, you may deplete your body of the others. People at risk for B-12 deficiencies include vegetarians who consume no animal products. B-12 is not found in many plants except for seaweed, alfalfa and hops. It is not certain how well B-12 is absorbed from plant sources either. The best sources are liver, eggs, clams, herring, mackerel and dairy products. The vitamin B family is very important if we want to maintain youthful function of the brain.

"B" IS FOR BRAIN
"Vitamin B Deficiencies and Misdiagnosed Alzheimer's"

As we age, the absorption of the B-vitamin group diminishes. This is why deficiencies are often seen in the elderly. Alzheimer's disease is not a normal part of aging. It is an unrelenting decline in mental function and memory loss due to the abnormal destruction of brain cells. Most often the first sign of this disease is short-term memory loss. The patient will remember who they went to high school with but forget where they were or what they did just that morning. Doctors and families should not jump to the conclusion that someone has this disease just because they are becoming forgetful. While the incidence of Alzheimer's increases with age, there is still no confirmation of the disease until after death. This is because that only upon dying is the brain able to be properly examined via an autopsy. What may be surprising is that a lack of vitamin B-12, (cyanocobalamin), may mimic Alzheimer's symptoms. People originally diagnosed with this disease were in fact found to have a B-12 deficiency. Once the lack of this nutrient was corrected, many patients returned to normal brain and memory function. Once again all of the B-complex vitamins should be included, but this is an example of how when even just one is lacking, adverse symptoms can occur.

B-1, (thiamin). Another B vitamin worthy of note is vitamin B-1 or thiamin. It enhances over-all circulation and also helps brain function and cognitive ability. Acting as a powerful antioxidant, it protects the body from the degenerative effects of aging. For example, Beriberi is a nervous system disorder and is caused by a lack of B-1. The components of your central nervous system include the brain and spinal cord, which are directly effected. Hence forgetfulness, nervousness and poor coordination all add up to symptoms often associated with old age and Alzheimer's disease.

Niacin or vitamin B-3, (riboflavin) This B-vitamin also helps in the function of the nervous system. Niacin lowers cholesterol and increases circulation. Therefore it is quite useful for patients with schizophrenia and other mental illnesses. Niacin is also an excellent memory enhancer. If you have diabetes, glaucoma, gout, ulcers or liver disease, you should use niacin only under the direction of your doctor.

Vitamin B-6 or (pyridoxine) is required by the central nervous system to operate at its best. It is needed for normal brain function for both young and old. Remember that absorption of all B vitamins may diminish as we age so we need to be vigilant to make sure we are including them in our daily regimen.

Choline is necessary for the rapid transfer of nerve impulses from the brain through the central nervous system. Without this B complex component, brain function and memory retention is severely impaired. Choline is primarily found in soya lecithin along with the other phosphorus- containing fatty acids inherent to this compound. Still, you can purchase a Phosphatidyl Choline Complex of 1300mg per capsule. This is triple the strength of the usual lecithin concentrate capsules. Lecithin makes the myelin sheath of nerve cells and facilitates their transmission of signals from one cell to the next. This is perhaps the best recommendation for preserving and even improving brain function as we age.

Perhaps the best advice is to choose a natural vitamin supplement, (most are coal tar derivatives), that is food based. Rainbow Light has a very good line that I have used for years and their products seem to break down easily. Products in gelatin capsules are often better than a hard-pressed tablet. This is because a gelatin coating will dissolve more readily in the stomach than a hard pill. Look at the bottle before you buy. Two piece gelatin capsules are what I use in my Natural Pharmacy course. The students learn to combine their own herbs, food enzymes and nutritional powders to make their own dietary supplements. Very empowering!

Here is a simple recommendation to build the basics of a vitamin program without going broke. Your primary supplement will be your multivitamin. Then you can build around that with other supplements that are often not available in a high enough amount in your multi's.

Recommended Daily Vitamins:

Balanced B-Complex Supplement, (should contain all of the B-Complex vitamins)

500 mgs of Esterized Vitamin C

400 I.U., Natural Vitamin E, or d-alpha tocapherol (May temporarily increase blood pressure when first used)

Daily Natural Food Based Multivitamin without Iron

C h a p t e r   3

YOUR AGE DEFYING HERBS
"Herbs for Health and Longevity"

■

GINGKO BILOBA FOR A LOT MORE THAN JUST MEMORY!

Gingko Biloba has captured the public's attention as the remedy for poor memory and mental acuity. You see young executives touting that Ginkgo has given them a mental edge for better performance on the job. The truth is that for most people under the age of 65, gingko offers diminished returns as to increasing blood flow to the brain. This is because under age 65, most adults' blood flow is quite sufficient. You will not see a noticeable drop off until after age 70 in most people! Younger adults can still benefit from the antioxidant qualities of Gingko. The gingko tree, or maidenhair tree, is very popular in urban areas because of its tolerance to smog and air pollution. The same antioxidant qualities that allow it to survive in such toxic environments make it quite appropriate for that application in humans. The following herbal blend combines Gingko in a synergistic formula rich in antioxidants and brain boosters that are sure to wake you up in the mornings:

Senior Brain Power Blend

1/2 cup dried Basil
1/8 cup of dried Rosemary
1/4 cup of dried Peppermint Leaves
1/4 cup of dried Gingko Leaves

Grind the dried leaves together until fine. Place in a teaball and steep in one pint of freshly boiled water for 3-5 minutes.

The peppermint stimulates the brain while the basil and rosemary heighten mental function and mental alertness. Rosemary is also a fantastic antioxidant, protecting the brain cells from the ravages of naturally occurring free radicals. It is a wonderful aid for memory retention. Just do not use it at night, it will keep you wide-awake! To this protocol, you might substitute a standardized Ginkgo Biloba concentrate for the dried gingko leaves. This may be taken with or without the tea. However, once again stay

Leaf of the Gingko Biloba Tree

away from the herbal tablets of Ginkgo. They are often too hard to break down for absorption. Try purchasing Ginkgo in two piece gelatin capsules or even sealed soft gels. They will break down much more readily for assimilation in the small intestine so you will actually get your money's worth.

A standardized product means that a certain percentage of the bioactive components of that herb are guaranteed in each bottle you buy. Some herbalists believe that this is not very important and that using the whole herb is. There may be something to this. Herbs are so very complex that we can not really choose only one chemical component from the plant and say, "this is the part that works". We can, however, make an educated guess and make sure the product has these bioactive components in addition to the whole herb. Here you have the best of both worlds and a more complete herbal product. To support this, many studies on the age defying effects of Gingko on the brain and body are done using GBE or Gingko Biloba Extract. It is easier to chart consistent laboratory results when the more uniform Gingko Biloba Extract is used.

GINGKO FOR MALE IMPOTENCE
"Helpful in Male Erectile Dysfunction"

Gingko does a lot more than increase blood flow to the head and provide antioxidant protection against free radicals. A study published in the Journal of Urology showed Gingko helps relieve impotence caused by narrowing of the arteries that supply blood to the penis. Sixty men with erection problems caused by impeded penile blood flow were given 60 milligrams of gingko a day. By the end of the year-long study half of the men regained erections. According to pharmacologist and author, Varro Tyler, "...there is an impressive body of literature attesting to the effectiveness of Gingko Biloba Extract, (GBE) in treating aliments associated with decreased cerebral blood flow, particularly in geriatric patients. These conditions include short-term memory loss, headache, tinnitus, depression and the like. Both clinical and pharmacological studies have shown that Gingko Biloba Extract promotes vasodilatation and improved blood flow in both the arteries and capillaries. There are also indications that it is an effective free radical scavenger. Large doses are required, which explains why a concentrate is used rather than the herb itself." Tyler goes on to state

that the commonly used form is a concentrated extract, standardized to 24% flavonoids, and 6% terpenes.

Herbalist Michael Hoffman cites research that shows
Ginkgo benefiting the normalization of blood pressure in the
circulatory system. It appears that Gingko reduces the tendency of clot formation in veins and arteries, suggesting use
in the prevention of coronary thrombosis and in recovery from
strokes and heart attacks. It has been shown to have lowered
blood pressure and dilated peripheral blood vessels in patients
recovering from thrombosis of blood clots. If you are currently
on Coumadin therapy you may soon see Gingko Biloba Extract take center stage for both thrombosis prevention and
blood pressure normalization.

HAWTHORN BERRY FOR HIGH BLOOD PRESSURE & HEART DISEASE
"Natural Help for Your Heart"

Looking at another factor that is accepted as part of getting
older is the onset of high blood pressure. Practically every
medical book will tell you that as we get older, the arteries
begin to become coated and the lumen, or inner diameter,
grows smaller. This constricted passageway does not allow the
artery the normal flexing ability; therefore blood pressure will
increase. Many blood pressure charts therefore allow for this
by citing normal blood pressure for a person aged 70 can be as
high as 166/91. The focus is all wrong here. Why don't we
question how the arteries got occluded in the first place and
if so, what can be done to regain normal function to them?
Scientific research into diets high in saturated or animal fat
has indicated that food choices most decidedly are the cause.
In any event, no matter what has happened in the past, you
have the opportunity to turn things around...today. An herb
that is proving to be a valuable ally in the fight against heart
disease and hypertension is Hawthorn Berry.

Hawthorn, (Crataegus species of the Rosaceae family), has been used for many years to treat heart failure in Europe. Active ingredients are extracted from the berries, leaves, and flowers and include antioxidants such as quercetin and rutin.

Studies done in Czechoslovakia, the United States and Germany suggest Hawthorn may benefit heart health on many levels. In lowering blood pressure, Hawthorn acts by dilating the peripheral blood vessels, moderating heart rate and by mild ACE, (angiotensin converting enzyme), inhibition. All of these add up to less stress on the heart and coronary arteries. Patients with New York Heart Assoc. functional class II, (mild to moderate), heart failure were given a daily dose of 600mgs of Hawthorn extract. After an eight-week period, study patients showed marked clinical improvement.

Caution should be taken, however, when using Hawthorn along with digitalis based heart medications such as Lanoxin (digoxin). This interaction may require a lowered dose of up to one half of the prescription drug. Hawthorn's benefits to the heart and blood pressure develop slowly over time. You need to remember that when using herbs potencies can vary from year to year according to soil and growing conditions, rainfall levels, and storage before processing. Standardization therefore becomes quite desirable. However, some of the best herbal products come from plants that you have grown fresh yourself. You are using the whole herb with all of its constituents and complexities.

Growing herbs yourself can be gratifying as even people with "brown" thumbs often find themselves having great success! After all they are only "weeds" and highly competitive in reproducing in the wild. Therefore, you should find them quite easy to cultivate in a sunny window or patio box for your own use.

Recommended Daily Herbs:

Standardized Gingko Biloba Extract, (Do not use if you are

taking Coumadin, aspirin or other blood thinners)
Standardized Hawthorn Berry Concentrate, (Use only under your health practitioner's care)

*****Caution!*** *Avoid Iron Supplements or Multivitamins with Iron unless recommended by your doctor!*

Chapter 4

Consumer Safety Tips
for Purchasing Herbs

■

Since the beginning of man's history, the quest for exotic herbs and spices has launched explorations of uncharted seas and lands. The ancient spice routes through Saudi Arabia, India and China bear witness to a way of life built upon the procurement and transporting of fragrant botanicals. Even in our 20th century, many exotic herbs and spices hale from the earth's four corners while others have been adapted and grown here in the United States. For example the oriental herb Ginseng has three major varieties including Japanese, Korean and American. The American Ginseng is considered superior the world over and even the Japanese have eagerly imported American Ginseng since the 1950's! Several factors make the same herb more desirable from one country or region over another. Soil conditions, rainfall, agricultural and processing practices all weigh in, to either add or detract from the herb's value and potency.

Ancient Chinese herbal medicine is quickly becoming integrated into western herb use and application. With a history that is reputed to date back more than 5,000 years, Chinese medicine is getting a second look today. In some aspects, this medical system was more advanced than those of Europe, with the Chinese establishing the circulation of blood close to 2,000 years before the West. By the 7th century AD the Chinese had been able to recognize diabetes and by the 10th century, they were successfully inoculating against smallpox.

Herbal medicine of the ancient Chinese included opium, rhubarb and cinnamon bark but also indicated the use of toxic metals such as mercury and arsenic. The use of mercury carried over into our 18th century, with Western medical doctors using it for practically every illness. Its use even contributed to the untimely deaths of King Charles II in 1685 and George Washington in 1799.

Today, traditional Chinese herbal formulas can still be purchased but since the names are in Chinese, consumers should be aware of some of the components present in these blends. For example gecko (Gejie), silk worm excrement (Cansha) and tiger's bone (Hugu) are commonly blended with Asian herbs as they are thought to add "therapeutic" benefit to the formula. In fact, 48 young American women developed kidney failure after using a Chinese herbal therapy for weight loss. The herbal preparation was suspect of having contaminants that accounted for this.

The growing and processing of herbs in the United States, while still unregulated, may have several advantages over herbs imported from other countries. For one, American herb manufacturers often employ standardization that offers a certain amount of quality control over their herbs. Through standardization, a certain percentage of the active ingredient(s) in an herb can be guaranteed in every bottle purchased. In Japan's Toyama Pharmaceutical University Hospital, fresh herbs from around the world are collected and analyzed. They have found big differences in the amounts of active ingredients present in the herbs tested depending on the climatic and soil conditions where they were cultivated. This is why standardized extracts are most frequently used in clinical assays involving herbs and are recommended above other forms in this book.

Consistency is important in scientific testing and it should be to you if you are seeking the therapeutic benefits reported by laboratory research.

Another problem cited by the university was that of mislabeling. According to their findings, herbal preparations do not always contain what their labels claim. The Canadian Drug Reaction Monitoring Program reports of adverse reactions due to heavy metals such as arsenic, lead, mercury and cadmium as well as prescription drugs phenylbutazone, aminopyrine, prednisone, testosterone and the sedative drug diazepam, (Valium) having been found present in dietary supplements imported from Asia (primarily China).

Overall, imported bulk herbs are perhaps the greatest offenders in this category. Often pesticides long banned in the United States are sold to and used freely by Third World Countries struggling to survive. Since bulk imported herbs are often not even checked for presence and levels of pesticides, there is no way to know if the product is contaminated.

As a consumer you can protect your health by carefully choosing your herbal preparations. Here are a few buying tips:

1. Look for both the common and Latin name on the label. For example Nettle is the common name and Urtica dioica is the Latin name telling you the genus and species.

2. Look for standardization. A certain percentage of an herb's active ingredient(s) can be uniformly standardized to insure that you get this same amount with every purchase.

3. Seek professional advice. Your local pharmacist may be of help, but for more personalized information it might be best to schedule a consult with a qualified health professional to discuss your specific health conditions and medications before taking herbs. **(Read more about this in the informative articles section of Dr. Miczak's Apothecary Website at: click-on.to/apothecary.)**

Certain prescription drugs can interact violently with many herbs so one must be careful while on such a medication program to evaluate any potential interactions ahead of time. If you have a health condition such as diabetes, epilepsy, high blood pressure, heart arrthymias or are pregnant, you need to be especially concerned about using herbs indiscriminately.

Even if you are perfectly healthy, there are certain herbs that can be dangerous for anyone to use. Here is a list of some of the most notorious along with safer herbal alternatives:

- **Use caution when using Dong Quai** (Angelica sinensis) Although recommended for PMS and menopausal symptoms, this Chinese herb's essential oil contains safrole, a known cancer-causing chemical banned by the FDA as a food additive. It even has the potential of causing miscarriage. Instead Use: Chasteberry (Vitex agnus-castus). "My patients say chasteberry eases breast swelling and tenderness," says Connecticut Gynecologist, Michael O'Reilly, M.D. As an added benefit it also helps to ease menopausal symptoms such as hot flashes, night sweats and anxiety.

- **Do not use Ma Huang** (Ephedra Sinica). Also known as Chinese Ephedra, it is used primarily for weight loss and energy. This herb weakens the adrenal glands, effects the nervous system like an amphetamine and likewise can make the heart race, increase blood pressure, cause mental confusion and insomnia. Instead Use: Chitin derived from shellfish for weight control. It has no CNS stimulants but will bind to excess fat from your food before it can be absorbed.

- **Do not use Comfrey** (Symphytum officinale) Although Comfrey is not absorbed through the skin it has been long touted as a wound healer. When large amounts are taken internally, problems such as liver disease have been reported. Instead use: Marigold creme (often sold as Calendula). It has antiseptic as well as antifungal properties making it excellent for all kinds of cuts and scrapes.

There are many other herbs that should only be used short term or under strict supervision such as hawthorn berry, echinacea and goldenseal. Remember each person is unique with varying degrees of body fat, differences in age, sex and metabolic factors so a therapeutic dose for your neighbor may well be toxic for you. A personalized evaluation taking into consideration these vast distinctions should be done before embarking on any such alternative therapy.

Arsenic and mercury (which have been found in a number of imported suppliments) are highly poisonous even in small amounts as they accumulate in the system over time with repeated exposure. Lead can cause lethargy and slowing of mental function and retardation, especially in children. Children who fall victim to lead poisoning must undergo chelation therapy.

Adding to the dilemma is the problem of misidentification, which is seen more often with imported herb products as previously cited. One such instance, occurring in May of 1997, turned up Digitalis lanata in a sample of raw herb product mislabeled as "plantain". Plantain is a common weed-herb and is highly nutritious as well as quite harmless. The mistake was traced back to some inexperienced herb gatherers in Europe who confused the two plant's identities. Nonetheless it had been sold under its mislabeled name for close to a year before it was voluntarily recalled, but not before causing a young woman to develop a serious heart block.

This should not dissuade one from using herbs, however. Yet like anything else, *"caveat emptor"* or "buyer beware" applies! This is the greatest argument to date to use herbs native to your home and grow your own as I have detailed in my book, *Nature's Weeds, Native Medicine...Native American Herbal Secrets* published by Lotus Press. This book includes a chapter with an herbal planting chart, gardening and herbal harvesting tips. You will have the peace of mind knowing that there are no adulterants in your freshly picked herbs that you will use for yourself and your family.

Chapter 5

ADDITIONAL DIETARY FOOD SUPPLEMENTS
"Putting it All Together"

■

These food supplements can be added to the diet to fully personalize the addressing of your needs. Women have specific health concerns for the phases of our reproductive cycle. Men have other issues. Some we may share as we get older and others will be specifically associated with our gender. That withstanding, you will find this chapter to be especially useful in mapping out *your* specific nutritional program. Consider this your fine-tuning section!

WHAT ARE FOOD SUPPLEMENTS?
"Supplements to Include on Your Youth Restoring List"

Food supplements fall into a class somewhat all their own. They are neither vitamins, minerals nor herbs. Still they offer quite a bit by way of nutritional value in augmenting the diet. For example, something such as wheat germ is actually the best part of the stalk head. It contains vitamin E, B-complex, magnesium, calcium and phosphorous as well as many other trace minerals. Raw wheat germ is best because heat has not destroyed any of its nutrients. You may also purchase capsules of wheat germ oil. In any case it is a food supplement because it has been derived from a natural food source. Products in this category are easier to assimilate, digest and absorb. After all, they are foods!

So you might wish to add this category of "nutritional helps" to your repertoire, as they are indispensable for building health quickly and naturally. Many can be incorporated into drinks, meals and dishes without much notice of flavor. Yet, you will truly benefit from their use.

The food supplements suggested here are easily incorporated into your daily routine. For example, the *Flax and Blueberry Frappe* can be made in a double amount and served two consecutive mornings. Most of us have trouble with compliance with a new routine. This will save you time in having to mix it fresh each morning. Simply shake the stored portion before serving. Liquefied food supplements have the advantage of getting into the digestive tract and thus into the bloodstream quicker. That is why something such as the *Blueberry & Flax Frappe* will give you instant energy without taxing your digestive tract. You know the feeling when you have eaten something just a little too heavy. That groggy weighed-down sensation. This is due to the enormous amount of blood, enzymes and energy being shunted to the process of digestion. This is a major energy draw that shifts blood from other vital organs such as the brain. The best way to wake up is with something light, digestible and packed with nutrients. Add a hard-boiled egg and perhaps a small, ripe banana as you are heading out the door and you have downed a potent breakfast-to-go!

Brewer's Yeast or Nutritional Yeast:

Food supplements such as cheese flavored brewer's yeast used in the *Way Mac-Macaroni & Cheese* lunch entree are a sneaky way to get even picky husbands to enjoy the benefits of this power packed product. Loaded with B-vitamins and amino acids, protein accounts for 52% of its total weight. Brewer's yeast, which is also known as nutritional yeast, is grown on a variety of media that will effect the flavor of the resultant product. For example, most brewer's yeast is grown on hops, which has a bitter taste. This is what gives brewer's yeast its characteristic flavor. Sweeter varieties are grown on blackstrap molasses and may be more palatable. There is a Swiss liquid nutritional yeast product that has been around for years. It is called Biostrath and I personally tried it and found it to be, "not bad". Its taste is more acceptable because it is made of malt, honey and herbs. Malt in and of itself is very rich in B complex vitamins and will sustain your energy at high levels for hours. Nutritional yeast boosts both your mental and physical energy. You may find yourself getting more done in less time and with less effort when using this supplement.

Essential Fatty Acids... The Fats of Life:

Essential Fatty Acids make up the necessary fats that the body cannot produce on its own. Hence the name "essential". They must be consumed in our foods to maintain health. The need for essential fatty acids are many. Often aliments associated with the elderly are actually marked deficiencies in essential fatty acids. Essential fatty acids can help with improving the appearance of skin and hair, prevent arthritis and lower cholesterol and blood pressure. Having enough essential fatty acids, or EFA's, in the diet can even help prevent a blood clot from forming. This is very important because when a blood clot forms in the arteries serving the brain, you end up with a cerebrovascular accident or stroke. When a clot forms in one of the vessels of the heart, you have a cardiovascular accident or heart attack. Either way what happens is tissue death because oxygenated blood can not reach those organs. Not everyone is able to take blood thinners. Those with bleeding ulcers would be one class of patients. This nutritional supplement offers much more than just prevention of clots, as you will see.

EFA's are found in large concentrations in the brain. Why is that? Well, these essential fats aid in the transmission of nerve impulses speeding them through the central nervous system. Without them you may experience difficulty learning or even recalling new information. Remember that this is one of the signs of early Alzheimer's? How many people have been misdiagnosed with this dreadful disease and even institutionalized when perhaps the cause was a deficiency in essential fatty acids. In any case the addition of EFA's in your diet will be one of the best investments in helping to turn back the aging clock that you can make. There have been studies using school children to see if EFA's would increase their ability to learn and score high on tests. Study participants had 1 tablespoon of flaxseed oil mixed in their yogurt or cottage cheese each morning. The results? After 2 weeks the teachers noted a great improvement in the student's ability to learn and retain new lessons.

This should be no surprise. A mother's own breastmilk is rich in EFA's. This "brain-fat" may account for breast-fed babies scoring a bit higher on their IQ tests than their bottle fed counter parts. Infant formulas still have not managed to copy the uniqueness and complexity of mother's milk. Instead of being enriched with essential fatty acids, formula manufacturers use cheap palm or coconut oils for the fat constituent. These oils are far inferior to the EFA's found in human milk and do nothing to support optimal brain growth and function. Some things of nature, man just cannot improve upon!

The two categories of EFA's are split into two groups. They are the Omega-3 and the Omega-6 EFA's. The Omega-3 branch of essential fatty acids can be found in our previously mentioned flaxseed oil, fish oils, walnut and canola oils. The Omega-6 oils are present in raw, (not roasted) nuts, seeds and beans. Omega-6 can also be found in borage, grapeseed, sesame, soybean and the most expensive of all, primrose.

Whichever type you choose, be sure to use cold pressed oils and NEVER use them in cooking. This is because heating destroys essential fatty acids and even creates harmful free radicals. Not what you would want from your vegetable oils.

Flaxseed oil is far and away my preferred essential fatty acid. One reason is price. The other reason is that is simply works so superbly. Studies using arthritis sufferers showed significant reduction in the pain, swelling and inflammation of arthritic joints. It can be purchased with or without the naturally occurring plant lignins, (fibrous part of the flaxseed). I favor the lignin rich variety but you may choose according to your own tastes. Just as was done in the study with school children, flaxseed oil should be mixed in a shake, cottage cheese or yogurt that contains a little fat. This allows the flaxseed oil to become emulsified into misciles or tiny oil droplets. Emulsifying the flaxseed oil in this way will assist in its absorption through the villi of the small intestine. Otherwise, if taken straight, it will act just like mineral oil resulting in a "lubricant laxative" with all its unpleasantries.

Evening Primrose Oil:

Evening primrose oil is perhaps the most costly of all the EFA's. The finest is said to hail from England and believe me, you will be paying the price for its airfare! It is used to help combat many problems assumed to be a part of old age. Thus evening primrose oil has been shown to help prevent hardening of the arteries or arteriosclerosis by lowering cholesterol, heart disease, multiple sclerosis and hypertension. It also helps relieve the pain of inflammatory diseases such as arthritis.

For women and men, evening primrose oil facilitates the release of sex hormones such as estrogen and testosterone. Women especially have discovered how well this oil works to quell hot flashes and vaginal dryness as associated with menopause. This is because, as previously mentioned, evening primrose oil promotes the production of estrogen. Not a bad thing unless you have an estrogen dependent cancer such as of the breast or uterus. Estrogen receptors in the tissues of these organs readily respond to estrogen and will begin to proliferate or multiply. This is why women in this category are often prescribed the drug Tamoxifen. This drug blocks the attachment of estrogen to the cells of the breast and uterus, preventing them from being activated into cancer cells. If you have breast or uterine cancer do not take evening primrose oil. Black currant or flaxseed oils are better choices. They are also less expensive.

THE SKINNY ON SOY
"The Benefits, the Risks"

Soybean production in the U.S. is at an all time high. Soy is used in animal feed, cosmetics, dyes, foods and beverages...the list just goes on and on. Women who are perimenopausal, (near menopause) swear by it for relief of menopausal symptoms. This is because of soy's documented phytoestrogen effects. Phytoestrogens are literally translated as "plant estrogens."

Now phytoestrogens are not to be dismissed as ineffective because they are derived from a vegetable source. Not at all! Phytoestrogens are much weaker than the endogenous estrogens (those made by our own bodies). All the same they are powerful enough to trigger the natural turnover of our own body's estrogen. This is preferable in many ways to estrogen replacement therapy especially if you are at high risk for developing female cancers. People in this category would usually be women with at least one first-degree relative who has had breast or uterine cancer such as your mother or sister. Therefore, use of phytoestrogens in lieu of estrogen replacement therapy might be a preferred method if these are your circumstances. *(see Chapter What a Woman Needs to Stay Young and Healthy)*

This brings us to the subject of soy. Soybeans (Glycinemax) are a member of the pulse family but are toxic if not prepared and processed properly. The many cultures of Asia figured this out over 5,000 years ago where soybeans have been used as a primary source of protein for at least that long. Right now, there are over 2,500 varieties in cultivation, some containing more protein than others. They yield even more than just a food crop. Soybeans are used in everything from inks to the making of plastics! Highly versatile, soybeans give us soybean oil, soy sauce, soy milk, tofu and is even used as a coffee substitute, but I would not toss the Folgers just yet. Still it is one of the best sources of phytoestrogens around. In fact eating just two servings of tofu a day, (8 oz of soy milk and 4 oz of tofu), has been shown to relieve hot flashes, lower cholesterol and even increase bone density. Soy is also the only vegetable that contains Omega - 3 essential fatty acids. These essential fats allow for the ease of synthesization or production of estrogen. An added benefit of soy is that it is suspected of helping to decrease the risk of breast cancer but *only if you do not already have it*. Keep this in mind and we will return to this point later.

The problem with getting the benefit of soy is in compliance. You will need at least 2-3 servings of soy per day to get the results described above. If you do not come from a culture that traditionally cooks with tofu, this might be hard to swallow, (pardon the pun). You might get around this problem by simply using a concentrated soy powder that can be blended into cereal, juice, milk or a shake as you will soon see. You will also need to take note of the fat content. Whole soy milk is very fattening, as many of my female clients / patients have already discovered. It is not unusual to see a gain of 4 - 5 % higher body fat after only two or three months on whole soy milk. So if you want your soy and to eat it too, make sure you choose the lower fat versions in both the milk and tofu.

Now the down side to soy. If you have already been diagnosed with a female cancer especially, **do not take, eat or use soy products**. It appears that something in the soy triggers the activation of preexisting cells. I have actually seen this happen several times in my own private practice. A woman with breast cancer will go through chemotherapy, medication, Tamoxifen, everything. She will finally go into remission and then say, "I hear tofu can help prevent breast cancer so I will start eating lots of it!" Wrong, wrong, wrong. Just as I have said before. Use of soy products may be of benefit *before* you develop an active cancer. However once you have it the use of soy may only work to reestablish it. One woman who came to visit me for a healthy eating program did just this. She was doing fine, but eating tons to tofu while in remission. Upon her next visit, the doctors noted her breast cancer had returned. The only thing that she had done differently with her diet was adding tofu. A sad lesson after all that she had been through, as she was back at square one. If this information helps but one woman, I have done my job.

Recommended Daily Food Supplements

Flax Seed Oil
Blueberries
Kelp, Dulse or Bladderwrack, Fucus or Seaweed
Brewer's Yeast
Soy

Chapter 6

DELICIOUS RECIPES USING YOUR RECOMMENDED FOOD SUPPLEMENTS

■

All right, this is where many of us fall off the wagon! We may have all the best intentions and be totally psyched for the transformation. Yet, without some practical guidelines as to how to reap the benefits from using the food supplements discussed in Chapter 4, you just may be going nowhere. This is because change may be good, but it is always hard. This chapter is designed to help ease you into that transition. Often times just remembering to take your vitamin pills is a challenge. Food supplements can help fill in the gaps because you do not have to think about taking them if they are blended in your everyday foods. How many of us forget to eat every day?

No one I know. So using food supplements as detailed in these delicious recipes will be a snap. You will even find defiant husbands who vow, "I'll never touch that healthfood stuff!" begging for seconds. Good nutrition like good food should be no sacrifice. These recipes were developed with the help of Marie A. Miczak, author and degreed gourmet chef. She has studied at Peter Kump's Culinary Arts School in New York City and writes internationally as a syndicated columnist.

First of all, every kitchen should have these basics. Once they are assembled, you will have no trouble whipping up these brain and body building treats in no time. Have the following on hand:

Blender or Food Processor

Dry and Wet Measuring Cups

Measuring Spoons

Whisk

Pyrex or Glass Cookware

Mortar and Pestle

These are the very basics and you will soon see that you do not need to spend a lot of money on fancy kitchen gadgetry that you most likely will not use. With a little organization you will find it easy to put together your morning routine for health. Now I am not going to bore you with the "you should know how important breakfast is" speech, which I am sure you have already heard too many times. The truth is that there is a knack to getting your body going in the morning without taxing your digestive tract.

A heavy traditional American breakfast of eggs, bacon, pancakes, fried potatoes, etc. is just too much for your stomach to handle right off the bat. This is because of the high amount of enzymes needed to break down all of these concentrated foods. What ends up happening is that so much blood and energy is diverted to the digestive tract just to begin to breakdown this super meal that it drains energy from other organs, such as the brain, in doing so.

In *Fit for Life* written in the 1980's by the Diamonds, they detailed this problem. Their solution was to eat only fresh, raw fruit until 12 noon. They promised weight loss and increased energy with this method. This was not a bad theory, although in practice many people may have a difficult time complying with the program. One variation on the theme that I see as a workable compromise is having a little fresh fruit as soon as you get up and then have my Blueberry & Flax Frappe as your breakfast entree. If you are still hungry, some scrambled egg whites with a few peppers added will set you firm. You are still able to have more concentrated foods, but here you are gradually adding them so as not to overwhelm the digestion process. The extra protein first thing in the morning helps keep blood sugar levels even and energy high well until lunch-time. You will find this working much better than a bagel or bowl of sugared cereal.

This is because simple carbohydrates, (refined flour products as opposed to complex carbohydrates), is converted immediately into glucose. This then calls for the release of insulin from the pancreas to allow the glucose access into the cells where it can be used as fuel. However once the excessive amount of insulin has been secreted to deal with the glucose derived from the carbohydrates, you may find yourself tired and sluggish.

This whole process is known as an insulin response and is most often seen in hypoglycemics, or people with too low blood sugar. A hypoglycemic patient will often present with very low blood sugar readings first thing in the morning. They also crave sweets and starchy foods since they make them feel better, but only for a short time. Once the over-killing amount of insulin is secreted in response to the large quantity of sugars and carbohydrates they have consumed, glucose levels "troth out" or dip below normal. The result is that the person is struggling for energy and has difficulty concentrating. So what do they often do to feel better again? That's right, they go back and eat more sweets and starches, which starts the whole cycle over again!

If this sounds like you, a low sugar, high protein alternative such as the Blueberry & Flax Frappe is the answer to your breakfast blues. There are so many good things about this power drink that it is hard to know where to begin! First ingredient is the fruit, those delightful blueberries. Low in sugar, rich in minerals including iodine, brimming with enzymes. Absolutely wonderful first thing in the morning. The flaxseed oil is next in the formula because it is rich in brain regulating essential fatty acids. The EFA's are also important to the normal production of female hormones, thereby moisturizing the skin from the inside out, keeping it smooth and young. The base or the liquid portion of the shake gives you a few choices. You can use rice, almond or soy milk. Rice milk has low allergy potential so it is good for people with food allergies and sensitivities. Rice milk does not have the same protein content as the soy or almond milks, so keep that in mind.

Next there is almond milk. This is made from pureeing almonds and extracting a "milk" from them that is rich, nutritious and high in protein, as are most nut milks. Almonds contain naturally occurring laetrile, the name given to the chemical amygdalin. Laetrile is also found in the kernels of apricots and peaches, both of which are also related to almonds. For many years, some scientists have seen laetrile as being a hopeful in curing cancer. Even though in 1981 the U.S. National Cancer Institute reported laetrile to be ineffective against cancer, patients who have actually survived cancer using this substance say otherwise. There is still a lot of debate and often times you will see organizations that accept huge donations from pharmaceutical companies downgrading a natural substance that cannot be patented.

The very last component in the Blueberry & Flax Frappe is barley and wheat grass powder. My personal preference for my client/patients is Phyto Complete because it is just that! Really you could alternate and just mix this powder in a little carrot or tomato juice for a nutritious change. It contains whole vegetable concentrates as well as chlorella, spirulina and barley grass among other high-energy ingredients. Since its flavor tends to take over, you might wish to serve it as I suggested in a vegetable juice rather than try to mix with soy, almond or rice milks. My choice for use in the Blueberry &

Flax Frappe however is a product called Kyo-Green by Wakunaga. This powdered mix contains barley and wheat grass powders, Bulgarian Chlorella, cooked brown rice and pacific kelp. All of these components are nutrient rich and will add quite an energy kick to your day. Combined in this super shake synergy, well, let us just say you might need to fasten your seat belt before drinking this! Now here is the brew:

Blueberry & Flax Frappe

1/2 cup of fresh or frozen Blueberries
1 cup cold Almond, Soy or Rice Milk
2 tablespoons Live Cultured Buttermilk or Yogurt
1 tablespoon cold pressed Flaxseed Oil
1 tablespoon Barley & Wheatgrass Powder
1 scoop of Soy Protein Powder
3-4 ice cubes

Combine all of these ingredients in your blender and puree. For an added variation you can add other fruits, but stick to blueberries or even strawberries, which are equally low in sugar if you are hypoglycemic. If you have normal blood sugar levels you might add a ripe banana to the blend. Bananas are not only loaded with potassium but they are rich in enzymes, which we need to break down our food.

The buttermilk or yogurt helps maintain a healthy intestinal flora. You will need to make sure the buttermilk and yogurt contain "live" cultures, though. Often times the label on the yogurt container indicates that the product contained live cultures before pasteurization. Once the product undergoes heat processing, it kills off the viable cultures, doing your intestinal tract no good. Look for yogurts sold in healthfood stores or purchase a yogurt maker and do it right. I used to make homemade yogurt for my children when they were small. It is quite simple and you can save a little from each batch that will serve as a starter for your next. You could not do that if the product had been heated to the point of killing the cultures.

In order to save time, you might wish to double the portion and save it in the refrigerator for the next day. This way you are not blending each and every morning. I just suggest that you not try to make this blend in too large of batches. Also, do not store for more than two days in the refrigerator once blended. It will not taste very good after a few days and the layers will separate out, making it difficult to re-blend into a homogenous liquid.

Always rushing out of the house in the morning? No problem. Get a thermos and pour away. You can take your drink on the train, bus or sip in a spill proof cup in your car. There is no reason why you cannot take it with you! Absolute and total nutrition on the go. This is an easy lifestyle adjustment anyone can make towards glowing health. What is even better is the fact that unlike vitamin pills, this drink is in a suspension. This means that in this liquefied form all of the nutrients are instantly available and totally digestible. This is why it will give you an almost immediate energy charge in about 20 minutes. What is even better is the energy lasts all day. You will not be hungry before lunch either, but in case you are, bring a hard-boiled egg or some low fat cheese with you. These extra protein foods will keep your blood sugar levels even and sustain you a bit better than a bagel or muffin. Remember, breads are starches and turn right into sugar in the body. If you are having trouble keeping your blood glucose up, then you will need to look at cutting back on both sugar and starch consumption since they are practically one in the same.

PLANNING MEALS FOR YOURSELF AND FAMILY

One of the biggest problems that faces women today is the fact that we truly still assume the responsibility of keeping everyone in the family happy. We try to keep the home clean, laundry ironed, shopping done, etc. often while holding down a full time job. As a result of constraints on our time, we may find ourselves getting take-out food more often than not. While fast food may seem like a lifesaver on a day that you just did not have time to defrost anything, it is no bargain for your health or your money. Each time you order out, you are missing an opportunity to build your health and after awhile, you will begin to reap the results. Low energy, weight gain and increased susceptibility to colds. Practically everything a healthy, well-nourished person doesn't have to worry about.

In order to make meal planning enjoyable and workable, you might consider enlisting the help of others who stand to benefit from your cooking. Those would be the people in your household you cook for. Elderly parents can chop and peel if they are able or even watch a pot or two. Younger hands can set the table and clean up the kitchen and dishes after meals. This way the whole cooking experience is not dumped on you because you now have help. I know it is difficult at first. Us women often want things done the right way, (ours)! We have to learn to let go of the minutiae of how the dishes are to be put away and the floor is to be mopped. They are really not as important as we think they are. In fact if you do not let younger and even older ones help out, they may begin to think that their contributions to the household do not count. Besides, you need help! Sorry to tell you this but "super mom" is dead. She went out with the 1990's. Women are learning that they must first take care of themselves before they can nurture others.

Having said this, you should also keep in mind the factor of time. What I am thinking about is wasting some time...together. What better place to do this than the family kitchen? This is the perfect place to slow down, catch up on the day's events and prepare a meal. You might even find that cooking can be therapeutic, not just for the nutritional value but for the calming effect that comes from focusing on creating something. See it as an outlet for both mind and body.

I would like for people to see that, number one, cooking does not have to be drudgery. Organization and getting the family to help out will go a long way towards removing this stigma. Number two, cooking is not women's work. We need to spread the responsibility for nourishing our families around a bit. We need to teach our children, especially, that they must make the proper food choices at home and in school if they want to feel their best. Otherwise, we become the "nags" of nutrition, constantly pushing healthy meals with little or no appreciation from those whom we serve. Believe me, anyone who is involved in the planning and preparation of a meal becomes that much more excited about the foods served and improving the quality of the menus.

Another common complaint when we strive to improve nutritional value is that of taste. Low fat is often equated with low taste while others balk at the thought of wheat germ and brewer's yeast. One way to get around this is to add food supplements to dishes that our families already enjoy. Mind you, you will need to use small quantities so as not to overwhelm the unwary taste bud. Still, you will be able to do a lot to improve the nutritional value of the foods you already serve, which may be a lot easier than changing the menu all together. The following recipes are examples of those types of transitions. Just by adding a small amount of these densely rich nutritional supplements, you will be increasing the food value of your meals dramatically. The first example is a delicious twist on the All-American favorite, Macaroni and Cheese:

Way Mac Macaroni & Cheese

4 cups of Macaroni Noodles
1 cup of Grated Sharp Cheddar Cheese
1 cup of Grated Munster Cheese
1/2 cup milk
1 tablespoon of flour

1/8 cup butter

1/8 cup Natural Nutritional Yeast

1/4 teaspoon of Sweet Paprika, (optional)

1/8 teaspoon of Hot Paprika, (optional)

Boil your macaroni until tender, drain and set aside. Melt the butter and begin adding the flour and then milk alternately with a whisk to avoid lumps. Add your grated cheeses gradually, mixing constantly to make your cheese sauce. (At the very last, add the 1/8 cup of Natural Nutritional Yeast to the cheese sauce.) Pour your cheese sauce over the macaroni, let stand for about 10 minutes and serve hot.

Variations on this recipe can be made by using a salsa cheese that is a little spicier, but then make sure to back off of the hot paprika. You won't need it. Also, you can boost the beta carotene and calcium levels of this dish by simply adding broccoli, which is rich in both of these nutrients.

Another food supplement that is so very good for you is wheat germ. Wheat germ contains vitamin E and B along with a balanced array of minerals, both macro and trace. Wheat germ is actually the embryo of the wheat berry and is similar to the chicken egg in being the embryo of the chicken. Nutrient dense, it is best raw and unprocessed. This is because heat diminishes its nutritional value. For this reason toasted wheat germ is the second best choice. Due to the toasting, it will last longer, but is not as good for you.

Raw wheat germ as well as toasted can be added to many foods without changing the flavor at all. In fact your family may come to enjoy the rich, nutty flavor wheat germ brings to many ordinary dishes. For example, when making meatballs or meatloaf, you might wish to substitute half of the Italian breadcrumbs the recipe calls for and use raw wheat germ instead. This way the flavor your family is accustomed to is still there, but with an added nutritional benefit from the wheat germ. Here is a great example adapted from the most delicious meatloaf you will ever taste, courtesy of my wonderful

Hungarian sister-in-law, Veronica:

Hungarian Style Meatloaf with Wheatgerm

1 lb. of 95% lean ground beef

1 16 oz can crushed tomatoes

1 tsp. malt syrup

1/4 cup grated parmesan cheese

1/8 cup Natural Nutritional Yeast

1 small onion, finely chopped

1/2 cup Italian style bread crumbs

1/2 cup Raw Wheat Germ

1 small egg

1/2 cup spaghetti sauce

1/2 tsp. salt

1/2 tsp. pepper

1 tsp. garlic, (minced)

1/2 tsp. Hungarian Sweet Paprika

Blend all ingredients together. I usually use a huge mixing bowl and a potato masher to help blend this mighty mass! Take your time for this step though. The secret to this meatloaf's success is that all of the ingredients are thoroughly blended so that the flavors completely permeate the meat. There are two methods of preparation as far as cooking the meatloaf. They are:

1. Turn the completely mixed meatloaf into a Crock-Pot that has been greased with olive oil.

Set the cook dial to high or cook all day on low, the choice is yours. Add a little extra spaghetti sauce to the top of the meatloaf before you place the top on the Crock-Pot. 1/2 hour before serving, you may add a little extra parmesan and mozzarella cheese to the top. Absolutely divine!

2. Place the meatloaf mix in an oiled glass Pyrex loaf pan, (you

may need to use two for this recipe). Cover the top of the meatloaf with a thin layer of spaghetti sauce and cook at 350 degrees. Once again, 1/2 hour before the end of cooking, add a little parmesan and mozzarella cheese to the top. Incredibly delicious!

Hungarian Meatballs, a Variation on the theme: You can make Hungarian Style Meatballs out of this same mixture. Simply brown the small meatballs in about a tablespoon or two of olive oil until golden brown. Next pop them into a crockpot of your favorite spaghetti sauce and let them cook all day. They are a great crowd pleaser and delicious enough to serve to company and guests.

So there you are. Your family will beg for seconds and you will be able to chuckle to yourself at how much your family loves "health food"! Now some people's taste buds are extra picky, so if your family can taste some of the nutritional supplements you have added to this dish such as the nutritional yeast or wheat germ, simply back off a touch. You do not want to overwhelm them with change, just gradually introduce it. You can always increase the amount later as the family becomes accustomed to the new flavors, which most likely they will come to enjoy once given a chance.

Essential fatty acids are total brain food. Trouble is many of us may be missing delicious meals that are rich in them. I am talking about a change of pace such as a salmon salad as opposed to the usual tuna salad, (bor-ing)! Salmon has far more essential fatty acids than tuna, which has some EFA's, but has to be monitored for high levels of mercury. Instead you can also add mackerel, herring and sardines to the list of deep-water fish that are rich in Omega-3 essential fatty acids.

These are all rich in the EFA fish oil because they have a higher fat content than, let's say, flounder. For example, a mere 4 ounces of salmon contains up to 3,400 milligrams of essential fatty acids, specifically Omega-3. The same four ounces of a fish with less natural fat such as flounder only has about 300 milligrams. Now which one would you choose?

Try to include more of these in your diet and you will reap the benefits beyond measure. Remember how your mother always told you fish is brain food? The proper type of fish such as just described is what she was really talking about. If you do not believe what Mom says, just keep in mind that a deficiency of essential fatty acids can contribute to an inability to learn new information and remember what you have already learned. Here is a great recipe that perhaps Mom never thought of!

Sumptuous Salmon Salad

1 - 16 oz can of Red or Pink Salmon

1 small onion finely chopped

10 black and green olives finely chopped

1 tsp. of sweet relish

2 tbs. of celery finely chopped

3-4 tbs. Soybean Oil Mayonnaise

Lettuce and Tomato garnish, (optional)

This is a delicious change from the ho-hum tuna salad. Rich in Omega-3 essential fatty acids you need only a 4-ounce serving to get a whopping 3,400 milligrams of this nutrient. If you would like, you can combine tuna up to 1/2 the recipe. This way you will have somewhat of a familiar flavor but still be on your way to improving your diet with a food so rich in essential fatty acids. This Sumptuous Salmon Salad is therefore good for your heart and brain.

Another variation on this theme is my mother's most excellent salmon cakes! Now before you think about getting out the icing and sprinkles, salmon cakes are closely related to crab cakes. My Native American ancestors enjoyed many such seafood delicacies and invented cooking methods such as clambakes and recipes for fish cakes of all kinds. Salmon was plentiful among my tribe's hunting grounds, so I can remember it being served my grandmother and mother as part of our traditional ethnic cuisine. They must have had widespread appeal as my father, mostly of English and Irish stock, enjoyed them too! Here is Mom's recipe:

Mom's Native Salmon Cakes

1 can of pink or red Salmon, (low sodium is available)

1 egg

1 small onion finely chopped

1/4 tsp. Old Bay Seafood Seasoning

1/8-cup bread crumbs

1/8 wheat germ

1/2 cup shredded, frozen hash brown potatoes

1/2 pound of shrimp, chopped

1 6 oz can of crab meat, (optional)

2-3 tablespoons of corn oil or canola oil

Combine all of the ingredients thoroughly. Heat your skillet to medium-high and add 2-3 tablespoons of corn, (original native recipe), or canola oil. Form the mixture into hamburger-sized patties and fry until golden brown. Make sure shrimp pieces are cooked until opaque, not translucent. Absolutely fantastic!

I hope you can see with the inclusion of these delicious recipes and drinks that taking a handful of pills everyday is not really necessary or in your health's best interest. Foods will always be better than supplements which, as I have previously alluded to, are often not even absorbed. Even if tablets do manage to break down, they may not be properly utilized unless there is a protein molecule for it to "piggy-back" onto. This is why it is most often recommended that you take your vitamins with meals. Chapter 2 expands on how to get the most out of what you spend on nutritional supplements. As we age, we often do not produce the hydrochloric acid needed to breakdown our foods. This is often more so the case with those who have an inability to absorb calcium especially because calcium, like most other minerals, requires a slightly acidic pH in order to become part of the bone's matrix or structure.

Chapter 7

EXERCISE TO LOOK & FEEL YOUNG

■

Perhaps the best thing that you can do for yourself is exercise. However, just like taking vitamins, we know it is good for us but compliance is always a problem. Weekend warriors who are for the most part sedentary for most of the week will often tackle heavy exercise and yardwork on their days off. This is a bad idea because suddenly throwing your body into work it is not accustomed to can cause soft tissue injuries as well as a shock to the heart that is not yet conditioned for such a strain.

Just as I have given you an example of incorporating food supplements into your daily menu, here I will show you how to incorporate exercise into your lifestyle, no matter what your level of training. I guarantee that you will save gas, have more energy, spare your joints and so much more if you simply invest some time and a little money into the following activities. Before we begin, here's the whole story:

EXERCISE, FOR EVERYONE!
Joint Sparing Aerobic Exercise for those with Arthritis or Wishing to Preserve Their Joints

If you suffer from painful arthritis, perhaps the last thing you want to think about is exercise. Just getting around can be extremely difficult, especially in the morning when stiffness is a problem for many. The truth is that maintaining tone, especially of the skeletal muscles, ligaments and tendons that support the joints is very important. Proper circulation and promotion of movement actually helps to keep the joints lubricated and healthy. The term arthritis really means inflammation of the joint, which is an accurate description of the disorder. As the collagen and cartilage covering the ends of our bones wears away, bones no longer glide against each other but grind down causing pain and inflammation. The result can mean damage to the tissues and nerves adjacent to that joint.

Analgesics such as ibuprofen that are commonly prescribed for this condition have their own drawbacks. First of all, they can cause sudden gastrointestinal bleeding. Secondly, they have been suspected of inhibiting the production of cartilage and collagen actually making the problem of erosion even worse. They may offer symptomatic relief at best but with a price. Now pharmacologists are saying that the newer brands of prescription arthritis products are no better than the older stand-bys' even though they are four times more expensive.

Certain exercises, however, are hard on even healthy joints and should be avoided. They include high impact aerobics, running and jogging, particularly on hard pavements and surfaces. The amount of pressure placed on your knees, for example, is increased sevenfold per square inch with each pounding step. This works to wear away the supportive cartilage that cushions the ends of the joints. This process occurs naturally as we age but is accelerated by such activities as just described and even from being slightly overweight.

Some may feel that they are in a "catch 22" situation here. In order to maintain joint mobility and ideal weight, they know they must exercise, but how? One would most certainly not want to exacerbate their condition and let's face it, it is really painful making the effort! There are a few ways around this problem that will allow you to get the cardiovascular conditioning and circulation of aerobic exercise but at the same time spare your poor joints.

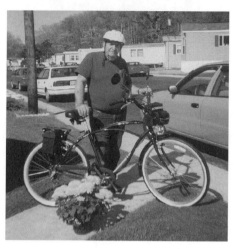

A satisfied customer with a Beach Cruiser with electric motor (contained in back-pack of bike) and stylish, essential helmet.

One form of exercise that is highly recommended is bicycling. The most efficient use of energy for motion known to man, there is practically no stress to the joints of the hips, knees and ankles, target areas for wear and deterioration. Indoor cycling or "spinning" has become a hot attraction at many posh gyms across the country and offers an alternative to cycling in inclement weather. All terrain bikes are also now very popular because they offer large tires, a comfortable seat and even shocks similar to what you would find on a car. All of these features cushion your ride and prevent your bones from being jarred. For more information on the sport of cycling, local trails, biking tips, cycling club links and driving directions to the store, visit MBC Discount Bike's official website at: www.mbc.genxer.net. If you are ever in central New Jersey, be sure to stop by MBC Discount Bikes, 898 Main Street, Belford, (part of Middletown), NJ 07748 or call (732) 471-1511.

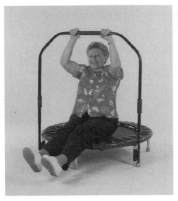
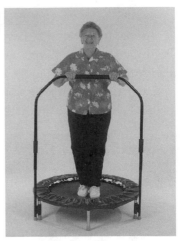

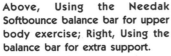
Above, Using the Needak Softbounce balance bar for upper body exercise; Right, Using the balance bar for extra support.

Another wonderful exercise is the sport of rebounding, or use of a mini-trampoline. Not to be confused with the department store "toys" that flooded the market during the 1980's, the professional quality rebounder is in a class by itself. I know about this first hand when I purchased a $29.95 model and proceeded to wear it out in no time. First some of the springs went, then the leather around the frame and on and on. When last seen it was put out for a yard sale because it became impossible to get replacement parts.

The professional breed of rebounder is epitomized by the industry standard, the Needak Soft Bounce. Just as the name implies, this rebounder is especially kind to your joints. You can run, jog or just bounce with out worry that you are doing further damage to your joints. In fact, the subtle changes in gravity experienced at the top and bottom of each bounce evidently have been seen to exercise the entire circulatory and lymphatic systems. The result is an energized body and mind with no knee creaks.

Needak, who also hosts an educational website on the sport of rebounding, provides an airtight warranty on their products, which are manufactured in America. One of their top units is their 1/2 folding mini trampoline that folds to resemble a taco and comes with its own carrying case. Being completely portable, you can take your unit outside, to the beach on vacation, etc. Retailing for around $240.00, it is a real bargain as you will get years of joint sparing aerobic exercise from it. Stop by the Needak website at: needak-rebounders.com or call (800) 232-5762.

All in all there are many factors that figure into joint health whether or not you have arthritis. Proper nutrition, perhaps even avoiding the nightshade family of vegetables, (peppers, tomatoes, white potatoes and eggplant) all of which contain the plant alkaloid solanine. Solanine is suspected of interfering with the muscle's enzymes therefore increasing pain and discomfort. Instead, include more sulfur containing foods such as eggs, asparagus, onions and garlic. Sulfur is key to the repair and maintenance of bone, cartilage and connective tissue as well as increasing the body's ability to absorb calcium into the bones.

As a final nutritional note, try eating fresh pineapple regularly. Fresh, (not canned or frozen), pineapple contains bromelain, a natural enzyme that helps in the reduction of inflammation of all sorts, including arthritis. Herbally, Native Americans have traditionally used willow bark for stiffness as cited in chapter 2 of "Nature's Weeds, Native Medicine...Native American Herbal Secrets". Similar to the bromelain found in fresh pineapple, willow bark also has the ability to arrest inflammation. In fact, acetylsalicylic acid, the chemical name for aspirin, was originally derived from willow bark and manufactured as this popular over-the-counter drug as early as 1899. Unlike aspirin, however, willow bark does not cause gastrointestinal bleeding as aspirin often can.

For more information on where to purchase books, audio and video tapes on walking, rebounding and cycling contact Collage Exercise Video Specialists at 800-708-9222 and order a free catalog. They offer a huge variety of exercise videos for every endurance level as well as formats to address the specific needs of those living with arthritis.

So you see, everyone should start now to preserve joint integrity. Most likely with the increased life expectancy, you will wear out your joints before the rest of your parts go! The 80's brought us high impact aerobics and the jogging craze. The 90's rung in the era of weight lifting at health clubs and gyms across the country. If you were born in the 1950's, well, you fit the baby boomer profile and more than likely have lived to experience all of this. See how things have changed, including life expectancy, since 1957!

In 1957...

The average yearly income was $4,594.00

A new car cost $2,157.00

A new home cost $12,225.00

A loaf of white bread cost .... 19 cents

A gallon of gas was only .... 24 cents

A gallon of whole milk cost $1.00

Minimum wage was .... $1.00 per hour

Life expectancy was 69.6 years as averaged for both sexes. American males are now at 71.5 years with American females coming in at around 78.2 years. We are living longer, but the question is what is the quality of those years? Medical technology has the ability to sustain a person who is no longer able to feel, breath or care for himself, but is that a desired existence for most of us? We all have our own opinions as to that subject, yet the common ground can be found in many people opting for homecare rather than institutionalization. I am speaking of "the nursing home." People in the marked phases of their life will look forward to the institution of attending public school, college and maybe even the military for training. However, how many people tell you they are looking forward to moving into a nursing home? Not too many. This is because this move signals the end of independence and self-direction. It is a hard pill to swallow, especially for someone who has grown accustomed to making his or her own decisions in life.

Loss of this privilege, along with freedom of choice, is often suspected of accounting for the high rate of senior depression associated with institutionalized seniors.

So the planning must begin now. Do you want to remain independent, perhaps living in your own home with assistance, or do you want to live in a nursing home for your final days? The personal health maintenance and planning you do now will often decide that outcome. Remember also that your children's lives are greatly effected, for isn't it one of them who most often has the unpleasant task of "putting you away". No child wants to do that. It is heart wrenching to say the least.

It was heart wrenching for me as my father could not be kept at home after a series of strokes left him severely disabled and paralyzed. He needs round the clock care that a visiting nurse could not provide. I remember the last day I spoke to him, when he was himself. He said, "Look after me now because Pop can't take care of himself." I have tears filling my eyes as I write this. Who knew that years of smoking, being overweight, stressed, aggravated and fighting through World War II would take its toll? My father was only 62 when he had his first stroke. While he was in the hospital under care for his first stroke, he began having seizures. It was horrible to watch. When I returned the next day after visiting him just the evening before, he looked right past me as if I was not there. He did not speak nor did he respond to my calling him. I was very unprepared for such a personality change, or should I say, loss.

Again, the care we take of ourselves is very important. In such a case as I have just described your children actually attend two funerals. One is when you are no longer the same personality due to a stroke or coma, the second is when death comes, perhaps prematurely because you bought into the fallacy that you were invincible. Do not become a sad statistic for yourself and your children. The time is now, "carpe diem," or "seize the day." It can mean so much, years later.

The next few chapters will break down what we need to stay young and healthy according to our gender. This information will allow you to fine-tune your own personal program to an even greater degree, so as they say...ladies first!

Chapter 8

WHAT A WOMAN NEEDS TO STAY YOUNG

■

If you are thinking, "A younger man," that is not quite what I had in mind here! While there is some correlation between greater longevity of people who are married as opposed to single adults, one thing is certain. No matter what your marital status, you can have an improved outlook on life and your health with a few changes in routine.

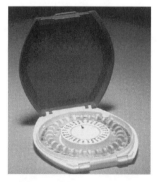

Woman who have used birth control pills years ago may find themselves at increased risk for breast and uterine cancer when opting for hormone replacement ther-apy later in life

Perhaps the biggest medication dilemma women face today is whether or not to go on estrogen replacement therapy as menopause approaches. There is so much controversy on this topic alone. Over the years we can see the correlation between women who have taken the pill and an increase in female cancers, specifically of the breast. Understandably this makes many women think hard before allowing their doctors to recommend HRT, or hormone replacement therapy, without adequate discussion. For example, a women with a first degree relative, (mother or sister), who has been diagnosed with breast cancer should really consider other options to HRT. This familial link to breast cancer already increases your risk as does age. The two factors combined should be weighed with great consideration.

This brings us to the subject of alternatives. What then is a good program of natural estrogen replacement, if such a thing is possible? First let us discuss what you are comparing the "natural" alternatives to. Perhaps the most bioavailable form of exogenous estrogen is Premarin. Otherwise known as con-jugated estrogens, this natural form is isolated from the urine of pregnant mares, hence the name Pre-MAR-in. This type of estrogen, unlike the uncogugated kinds, is easily absorbed by the gastrointestinal tract. Therefore, due to the chemical struc-ture, they operate just like normal endogenous, (produced by the body), estrogens. What are the benefits? Well conjugated natural estrogens have been shown to reduce hip fractures by 25%. This is due to the prevention of such fractures in main-taining bone mass, not by reversing osteoporosis.

Premarin also reduces low-density lipo-proteins, or LDL, otherwise known as the bad cholesterol responsible for laying down the arterial plaque that slowly occludes or narrows the arteries. By similar action these same conjugated estrogens increase your high-density lipo-proteins, also known as HDL's, or the good cholesterol, which helps remove accumulated cho-lesterol from the arteries. Lastly, one of the main reasons why women will opt for this form of estrogen is that Premarin in-creases cervical and vaginal secretions, keeping the tissues moist and thick. The problem of vaginal dryness effects more than just intimacy. Vaginal atrophy and dryness can invite increased incidences of infections in that area. The mucosal secretions form a barrier between the lining of the vagina and bacteria that may be introduced into the canal. There is a lot on the table here for discussion, but as with any medication protocol, you must also consider the down side.

Conjugated estrogens have side effects both long and short term. For purposes of illustration, I think it best to consider the long-term effect first. Use of estrogens increases your risk for developing breast, uterine and ovarian cancers, tumors of the liver, hypertension and blood clots. These are not just transient annoyances. They are all potentially life threatening, long-term health problems that you should carefully think about before embarking upon this form of therapy. The more minor side effects of estrogen are acne, breakthrough bleeding, fluid retention, headache, breast pain, nausea and vomiting. Do you see the difference in the two groups of side effects? However, they are all lumped together under adverse side effects in many pharmaceutical drug information printouts as if they are all merely temporary annoyances! Don't be fooled.

Also you will need to note the potential for drug interactions while taking conjugated estrogens. For example, you will need to avoid taking the immunosuppressive drug, cyclosporin. Cyclosporin is the generic name for Neoral, Sandimmune and Sang-35. This medication is used to treat autoimmune diseases, which is where the body turns against itself, and the immune system destroys crucially needed tissue and cells. Examples of autoimmune diseases include type I diabetes, (aka juvenile diabetes), rheumatoid arthritis and psoriasis. Cyclosporin is also indicated to prevent allograft rejection, which occurs when someone receives an organ transplant.

If you are on conjugated estrogens and take cyclosporine, the interaction could be quite serious. This is because the estrogens inhibit the metabolism of cyclosporin, causing high levels of the medication to accumulate in the tissues. This can lead to nephrotoxicity (kidney damage) and/or hepatotoxicity (liver poisoning). Likewise if you drink or smoke while on estrogens you greatly increase your likelihood even more so of developing serious cancers.

So where does this leave you? What sort of working alternatives do you have that will assist in increasing your bone mass, preventing heart attacks and keeping your skin soft, supple and moist even in those intimate areas? Well it may be easier than you think. God has provided us with an abundance of natural foods that contain plant estrogens clinically known as phytoestrogens. They are weaker plant analogs of our own hormones, but act in the body to help naturally facilitate the production of estrogen.

Just because you go through menopause does not mean that estrogen is no longer present or produced in your body. Yes your FSH, or follicular stimulating hormone, will begin to rise as estrogen production slows down but all is not lost. Your body simply shifts into "maintenance" mode during menopause. You begin to produce a weaker form of estrogen called estrone. Also, other organs that are part of your endocrine system begin to produce estrone for you as the ovaries continue to contribute less to this effort. It is this change or shift from the stronger estradiol that was once produced by the ovaries that causes the symptoms of hot flashes, vaginal dryness, insomnia and night sweats. Once the body adjusts, these symptoms will dissipate. Still you do not have to wait it out. There are things that you can and should do even if you are perimenopausal that may include a time span of up to ten years before you no longer have menstrual cycles.

By including some of the following foods in your diet everyday, you will give your body the building blocks it requires to assemble the female hormones needed to keep you young and strong:

- **yams,** (These are a different species than sweet potatoes and people often confuse them.)
- **soy beans,** (2-3 servings per day, for example 8 oz. of soy milk is one serving, 4 oz. of Tofu is another serving.)
- **red clover leaf tea,** (1 oz of dried herb to one pint of boiling water. Steep for 3-5 minutes and drink up to 2 cups per day.)
- **flaxseed oil** (up to 1 tbs. per day. Do not cook with flaxseed

oil as heat ruins its benefits. Mix in soy or almond milk, yogurt or cottage cheese made with a little fat for best absorption.)

All four of these foods are rich in phytoestrogens and are quite effective in picking up the slack when your own production of estrogen begins to wane.

Yams

Yams differ greatly from sweet potatoes. Yams are from the subtropical and tropical family Dioscoreaceae and can weigh up to 30 pounds each! The sweet potato, (Impomoea batatas) is actually a member of the morning glory family and is much smaller. Also, sweet potatoes are native to the new world tropics. Look closely at the labeling at the supermarket on fresh produce. Sometimes even they make a mistake. Yams are usually thicker, rounder and lighter in color than sweet potatoes.

Yams are great as an alternative to white potatoes. Nutritiously they have been used for centuries as a basic food staple in many tropical parts of the world. I can remember working in the Cook College Food Science Lab during the summer while I was in Pharmacy school. One of the graduate students was from Nigeria. He showed me his friend's wedding pictures from his country and pointed to the "gifts" brought by the guests. In the back of a pick-up truck, ten hands high were these yams, but unlike any I had ever seen before as they were each the size of a toddler! I had no idea that they grew that big. African Americans brought them to America when they came over as slaves centuries ago. Some of their recipes include making yams and collard greens, and sweet potato or yam pies that taste somewhat like pumpkin, (my personal favorite)!

Soy beans

Soy products come in many varieties. Tofu, tempeh, Miso, Edamame, Natto, Okara, and textured soy protein are just some of the variety of food products made from soybeans. The key plant estrogen isolates in soy are the isoflavones genistein and daidzein the symptoms of menopause such as hot flashes, night sweats and osteoporosis. In one clinical test, women who ate 45 grams of soy flour daily experienced a 40% reduction in menopausal symptoms. Similar to flaxseed oil, soy is the one of the few plant sources for the EFA, Omega-3 fatty acid. You will remember the Omega-3 are noted for their ability to reduce the risk of heart disease and cancer. Soybeans are also the only vegetable source known to have all eight of the essential amino acids, thus providing a complete protein. Soybeans are also rich in B vitamins and calcium. Here is a basic chart of amounts and comparisons, based upon 50-75 gms of soy protein per day, which is recommended for maximum benefit:

Soy Flour: 1/2 cup - 50 mgs

Soy Milk: 1 cup - 40 mgs

Tofu: 1/2 cup - 40 mgs

Soy Nuts: 1 oz - 40 mgs

Miso Soup: 1/2 cup - 40 mgs (caution: 1 tbs. of Miso contains 600 mgs of sodium!)

Tempeh: 1/2 cup - 40 mgs

In order to get the health benefits of soy you must eat it daily. Helpful soy compounds, such as the genistein previously mentioned, only stay in the body 24-36 hours at the most. Cells will quickly become depleted of this substance after less than two days of not eating soy products.

Note: If you have already been diagnosed with breast cancer, do not consume any soy products! For more information read Chapter 5, "The Skinny on Soy".

Red Clover, (Trifolium pratense)

Think of the purplish clover blossoms from which bees extract nectar to make honey. Sweet, fragrant, delicate. Red clover was mostly used in the past as a fodder crop for cattle. This is because it is naturally rich in vitamins and minerals. This same plant is also rich in phytoestrogens. During the 1930's red clover became a widely used anti-cancer remedy. Following this, red clover is still prescribed especially in Europe for breast, ovarian and lymphatic cancers. Its plant constituents include the isoflavonoids which, as previously discussed, are responsible for the estrogenic activity. You can make a refreshing summer tea or hot brew by steeping 1 oz of herb to one pint of water. Primarily, you will want to use the leaves as they contain most of the isoflavonoids. If you purchase the herb in bulk, however, most herb companies will include some of the sweet blossoms in the mix. Delicious! Red clover also has anti-inflammatory activities therefore it is also good for arthritic complaints, which is a disease of inflammation. Standard dosage for estrogen building help is 2 cups of infusion per day.

For more information on Red Clover and herbal preparations read *Nature's Weeds, Native Medicine: Native American Herbal Secrets* by Lotus Press.

Flax Seed Oil (Linum Usitatissimum spp)

I covered flax seed oil in Chapter 5 under the heading of Essential Fatty Acids...The Fats of Life. I also gave you a great recipe using flaxseed oil in Chapter 6, called the Blueberry and Flax Frappe. However, you should be aware of flaxseed oil's ability to facilitate the natural production of estrogen. Another name for flax is linseed; they are actually one and the same. Flaxseeds contain cis-linoleic and apha-linolenic acids. These essential fatty acids can not be manufactured by the body, but must be obtained from an outside source. The EFA's previously mentioned are necessary for the production of hormones like prostaglandins, (actually classified as autocoids), which are needed for many body functions. For instance, prostaglandins influence the breakdown of fat, fluid balance, blood clotting and flow, neurotransmission, function of the pancreas and the ovaries. Without essential fatty acids, the production of prostaglandins may be seriously hindered resulting in health problems relating to the organs and functions they serve.

Up to one tablespoon per day of flaxseed oil is recommended for proper maintenance of estrogen production. Take the flaxseed emulsified in a shake, yogurt or cottage cheese, just as long as it contains a little fat. Also you might wish to choose the lignin rich type of flaxseed oil. When you increase your essential fat intake, you will need to make sure you are taking enough vitamin E. These oils can go "rancid" in the body, therefore getting an adequate amount of antioxidant rich D-alpha tocapherol is imperative when adding them to your diet.

A Word about Osteoporosis and Hypothyroidism Medications

While the soy is rich in absorbable calcium and adding these phytoestrogen rich food supplements to your diet will help deter osteoporosis, you will need to be sure that you are still getting enough calcium. Women who have been on Synthroid, (levothyroxine sodium), for a number of years also run the risk of developing osteoporosis at a higher rate than the general population. I have seen relatively young women in their mid 50's with osteoporosis. Adding to this, when a women with a hypoactive thyroid goes through menopause, that phase of life automatically accelerates bone loss. Hence the combination of these two factors equate to increased incidence of spinal and hip fractures at a relatively early age.

How do you know if you are in this category? If you have been taking Synthroid or Armor Thyroid for over 3 years, then your own thyroid is most likely no longer producing its own thyroid hormones. This is part of the negative feedback mechanism of homeostasis. Simply put it means that when you introduce an outside source of a hormone into your body, the endocrine system acknowledges that by signaling the shut down of production from that target organ. In this case, your body senses adequate amounts of thyroxin in the bloodstream, so your own thyroid stops making its own and begins to atrophy or shrink. This is why once you begin this sort of medication, you will be on it for life. The news does not get any better when you go through menopause either. It appears that estrogen replacement therapy may not work very well because it competes with the same receptor sites as the Synthroid, displacing it. So combining Synthroid with hormone replacement therapy may require higher amounts of the thyroid medication to function normally. If this has happened to you, discuss it with your doctor or pharmacist.

In any event, whether on Synthroid or not, you might wish to review Chapter 2, Are You Boning Up on Calcium? The Best Type of Calcium for You and Your Bones. Once menopause is reached, which is the total cessation of your menstrual cycle, bone loss really picks up. If you are one who engaged in fad diets in your 30's and 40's, well, you may have to pay the piper now. Still, nature is forgiving. Did you know that you get a completely new skeleton every 8 years or so? That is about the average rate of bone tissue replacement. Your skeleton is a living structure, tearing itself down and then rebuilding again, but only if the right elements are present. Other factors can also effect the function and even shape of your inner framework. Did you know that if you habitually slouch, for instance, your spine will grow to follow that curve? Just the simple act of straightening yourself up and walking erect has wonderful effects on both your physical and psychological being. First it builds self-esteem and reflects to the world your confidence and youth. It also allows your lungs to fully inflate, oxygenating the blood, optimizing both physical and mental functions. So your mother's admonition to "Stand up straight and stop slouching," is well founded in medical science!

Since your skeleton is a living matrix of bone tissue, it must be properly fed to maintain proper functionality and strength. The amount of calcium that a woman needs during menopause is debatable only because various types of calcium have different bioavailability rates. The most common and cheap preparations contain calcium carbonate that is derived from rock! These are the seedlings for the formation of kidney stones. Sorry, but the body does not recognize a rock as a food source so you shouldn't either. People that have been recommended Tums as their calcium supplement have often been very sorry only a few years later when they had to undergo lithotripsy, or the breaking down of kidney stones via ultrasound waves. I do not know about you, but I can think of quite a few other places to spend my vacation days.

The current recommended amounts of calcium needed by postmenopausal women are between 1,200-1500 mgs of calcium daily. As mentioned previously, the amount you take and what you actually absorb may vary greatly.

Since no chapter on women's health would be complete without covering stress, the next article is also taken from my syndicated newspaper columns that are published by newspapers across the country and are even distributed abroad. We women internalize so much more than our male counterparts. From birth we are trained to be supportive caregivers, putting everyone's needs ahead of our own. While this level of selflessness is the stuff martyrs are made of, health-wise, it can account for women having far more stress and psychological related disorders than men. It should be apparent that in order to take care of others, we must first care for ourselves. I know that this may be a tough concept to sell, but it is absolutely true. You will find that you have much more to give to your family if you first invest in your own self-care on a daily basis. Your health depends on it, as you will see in the following article:

NATURAL STRESS RELIEF FOR WOMEN

Stress kills! Well perhaps not right away, but over time the wear and tear stress wreaks on our bodies is hard to deny. It is estimated by medical science that stress accounts for over 80% of all illness. Doctors even report that at least 75% of their office visits are stress related.

What exactly is stress and how does it effect us physically? Actually, stress is the fight or flight reactions that trigger our body's flow of hormones and chemicals that prepare us for battle or retreat. Either way, repeated stress chemicals in the bloodstream could make our immune systems weak and account for increased colds, respiratory infections, colitis and the progression of cancer. Likewise there have been links to stress as contributing to increased incidences of hypertension, heart attacks, diabetes, asthma, allergies and back aches.

Not only that but stress also depletes the brain of serotonin, an important neurotransmitter responsible for maintaining a positive mood. Other important brain chemicals are likewise depleted during the triggered fight or flight responses. This has been associated with the inability to remember things under stress. Temporary loss of memory function is therefore linked to stress.

Now the good news. There is a lot that you can do to control stress in your life as well as counteract its effects. Here are some sure-fire natural stress busters to try:

- Get enough complex carbohydrates. Do not get taken by the Atkins diet hype. Your body needs whole grains, which are rich in stress relieving B-Complex vitamins. In fact, eating a baked potato can bring up brain serotonin levels in as little as 20-30 minutes!

- Get at least 7 hours of sleep every night. Sleep deprivation is very common among us competitive Americans. By doing so you may be undermining your full potential for productivity for work and play if you do not get adequate sleep.

One study has shown those who received enough sleep every night lived longer. Now that is a real bonus.

- Limit your caffeine intake. This will in turn allow you to get your 7 hours of sleep every night. Not only that, but the caffeine found in only 2 cups of coffee can destroy your body stores of both vitamins B and C. Caffeine is a stress inducer in and of itself, making you jittery and addicted along the way.

- Do something relaxing for yourself each day. This falls into the category of self-care. De-stressing through reflection or prayer every day is a wonderful way to get in some quiet time for yourself. This can also be done in conjunction with other activities. For instance, imagine a warm bath at the end of the day scented with the aromatherapeutic benefits of lavender oil. Light a vanilla scented candle while reading a good book. If you make it a priority, this special time can keep stress out of your life. (For more information on the benefits of Aromatherapy, visit our special section headed by Marie A. Miczak, AIYS, Diplomate of Aromatherapy at: www.miczak.com)

Learn to get negative emotions off your chest by expressing them in a positive way. Open and honest communication is essential. The Bible has a wonderful admonition in telling us not to let the sun set with you remaining in a provoked state. It also has some excellent advice as to forgiveness and not giving ear to every derogatory thing people may say about you. In life, you are just going to have to let some things go. An unkind word from a neighbor, being slighted at not being an invited guest at a friend's house. Life is full of bumpy relationships made even bumpier when we over-react. On the other hand, do not concern yourself that people will not think you are "a nice girl" if you stand up for yourself either. Often times we just do not want to rock the boat or be accused of being difficult. Forget that! Simply speak up. Firmly, assuredly state your beef and what you need from the other person. The other person may even accuse you of being oversensitive, (a common destractive ploy). So what? Just as one of my favorite law professors says, "Keep your eye on the ball," and do not allow yourself to be sidetracked over comments on your behavior when the other person is really at fault.

I think lastly us women need to lighten up. Humor, wit and cracking jokes seem to be totally acceptable as part of male behavior but not for women. Well, you can change all that. People actually appreciate a good sense of humor. I am not saying go in for stand up comedy but telling a joke every now and then shows the world that you have self confidence and a mind. The physical act of laughing, even if at your own jokes, is extremely beneficial to the cardiovascular system and releases endorphins or feel-good hormones that help us cope with life's adversities. If you do not believe this I can tell you that when I donated my time to do free blood pressure checks for my town's street fair, the group with the best blood pressure and pulse rates were the performing clowns! One clown even tried to ask me for a date. (Sorry, but I always wanted to say that!)

Even though they were not exactly young men, (55-64 years old), their body fat, heart rate and blood pressure were closer to men 1/3 their age. Although it was a little difficult to tell under all that make up, they actually looked younger too. Since one of these clowns tried to ask me out to dinner, I assure you his hormones were functioning at about a 20-year-olds level as well! So the moral in all of this is to adopt an upbeat attitude as laughter is perhaps the best stress buster of all. You will also find that you are much more fun to be around too.

Chapter 9

WHAT A WOMAN NEEDS
TO LOOK YOUNG

■

All right, let me appeal to the vanity in us all. Let's face it, the image we project to the public reflects how we feel inside. Did you know that patients who come to the doctor's office with make up, freshly pressed clothes and their hair done are often made to wait longer? This is because you do not "appear" sick! Other more scruffy patients may easily be taken ahead of you due to the fact that you do not look as ill as the rest. Caring about how we look is more than just vanity, though. If you look at the mentally disturbed and depressed, they often have very little interest in their outward appearance. This is not normal because we humans are social creatures. A whole industry has grown up around our desire to look and smell good, adding to our convivial appeal.

THE LIPSTICK TEST

Far from being a clinical assay, the Lipstick Test is a name given to patients who are starting to "come around" after a bout of illness. Very sick women in the hospital will often neglect their appearance. They just do not feel well enough to care for these extra personal things. However, as she begins to feel better, she may ask for a hand mirror and yes...some lipstick! This is an excellent sign of her progressive recovery. The same philosophy goes for breast cancer survivors. They will many times lose their hair, healthy coloring and weight all due to the chemotherapy. It is really a low point for many women being so sick and having to watch vestiges of their femininity disappear. Hair loss for a woman alone is often devastating. The Nazi concentration camps shaved both men and women's heads for a reason. That reason was to make them feel vulnerable and weak. So losing our crowning glory is a reason for depression in and of itself.

That is why there are services and classes just to show women how to use wigs, make-up and prosthetic breast forms to make them look better. It is well known that when you look better, you will feel better. It is too soon to say, but it appears that increased survival rates for breast cancer patients may be correlated to women who availed themselves of these optional programs during treatment and recovery. Depression due to any source causes the immune system to break down, lessening your chances for healing.

SKIN CARE AS WE AGE

This chapter will give you some wonderful formulas for clear, smooth, moist skin at any age. If you are already entering menopause, keep in mind that diminished estrogen production will automatically effect the look of your skin. Most often you may notice a thinning of the dermis, the thicker layer under the epidermis. What this means is that less estrogen will cause less oil and collagen to be produced. So the outer layer begins to sag and not "fit" snugly the way it used to. This is why getting a face-lift may not solve all of your problems. It is the structure under the skin that also needs reinforcing.

Unfortunately, much of the hype about products that include collagen and elastin are just that. The molecules of these substances are just too large to penetrate the epidermis. They may have moisturizing qualities, but they cannot get down into the skin to do very much good where it is needed. You will find yourself paying thousands of dollars at the make-up counter for products that do little more than sit on top of the skin. This is not to say that nothing works. There are a few products and non-surgical procedures out there that give excellent results for less than you are paying at the Chanel counter.

Glycolic Acid Peels - This is an in office procedure that is less caustic than the stronger phenols, using concentrated fruit acids to slough off the top layer of skin and encourage new cellular growth from deep within. The result is smaller pores, smoother skin, diminished freckles and a luminous glow. This treatment will not remove deep wrinkles or creases, but fine lines virtually disappear. Dermatologists use a stronger percentage of the glycolic acid than salons can acquire. They also have more training to deal with reactions such as irritations and burns. While rare, these side effects can occur in

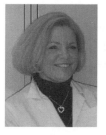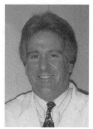

Jane Goldberg and Dr. Paul M. Goldberg offer Glycolic Acid Peels in a safe and clinical setting

sensitive patients. You do not want someone putting this kind of chemical on your face and then running off to check on another client's perm! Skip the salon, go to the dermatologist's office. One such plastic surgeon who offers this procedure at his Matawan, New Jersey office is Dr. Paul M. Goldberg. "These peels are effective in addressing fine lines and wrinkles. It is an excellent alternative to some of the more invasive procedures such as dermabrasion yet still offers smoothing and firming of the skin without the associated risks."

Generally the procedure starts with coming in once a week for 10 weeks for the mini-peels.

Once the skin has been conditioned, you need only keep a maintenance, having the peels done once every six weeks or so. The results are often just short of miraculous. A luminous glow, even skin tone, reduction of fine lines and wrinkles, tighter, firmer skin and a farewell to acne breakouts all in the same package. Incredible.

Natural Spa Treatments...for Pennies! - There are a few natural at-home facials that can be used based on the benefits of naturally occurring glycolic acid. These "fruit" acids are present in milk, sugar cane and many other edibles. Don't laugh. People spend top dollar to get such treatments that are all the rage at posh beauty spas across the country. Using fruits, essential oils and botanicals they offer a refreshing change of pace for both you and your skin.

So since you have been so good, I am going to share some of their pricey secrets for beautiful skin from head to toe. These are reprinted from *Secret Potions, Elixirs and Concoctions: Botanical & Aromatic recipes for Mind, Body & Soul* written by my daughter, (yes, I am that old), Marie A. Miczak.

Just do not blame me if you start speaking with a French accent, crave Perrier and demand winter trips to the Riviera: *Secret Potions, Elixirs & Concoctions* by Marie A. Miczak, Lotus Press.

EXCERPTS FROM CHAPTER 4: SKIN & BODY CARE

A great number of posh spas are now using "natural" and "botanical based" treatments. Some are even prepared fresh on site. The problem comes with the fact that many people do not have the funds to pay the ridiculous fees charged by some establishments. If they are able to pay, they can only afford to be pampered once or twice a year on special occasions perhaps. Some treatments need to be applied on a regular basis before you start to notice a real difference. Lastly, many people do not feel like, or have the time to, trudge into a spa for the whole day. To remedy this, many spas and cosmetic companies are now producing and marketing products to use at home. Unfortunately these products can be quite expensive as well and do not use 100% pure and natural ingredients. The only real way to know exactly what you are putting on your skin is to make the product yourself. Of course you can not make everything at home, but little by little you will find yourself replacing store bought items with the sensuously pleasing ones found in this book.

And now...the Formulas.

Body care

Honeysuckle Body Elixir

1-Cup fresh honeysuckle flowers

2 Cups spring or distilled water

1 teaspoon pure vanilla extract

In a small pot bring water to a boil, reduce heat to very low and add flowers. Turn heat off completely after 10 minutes. Cover and let stand on stove for 5 hours. When done strain off all plant material and place in a clean glass bottle. Use as an all over body mist or in clay masks. Keep all unused portions refrigerated and for no longer than a week.

Variations

Try these recipes for your specific skin needs.

Gentle:

1 Cup of fresh rose petals or 1/2 dried

1 Cup of water

Rose is extremely gentle for sensitive skin. Use after a bath for a real treat.

Refreshing:

2 Tablespoons of lemon zest

1 Cup of water

1 teaspoon of vanilla extract

This formula works great in the morning after a shower to help wake up your senses.

Moisturizing:

1 Cup of fresh rose petals or 1/2 dried

1 Cup of water

1 teaspoon of banana extract

5 drops rose essential oil (optional)

Placing body elixirs in mist bottles will make it easier for you to use and enjoy.

Amazon Rain

4 Cups spring or distilled water

1/2 teaspoon honey

10 drops of coconut fragrance oil or 2 teaspoons coconut extract

1/2 teaspoon pure vanilla extract

5 drops of jasmine essential oil

Mix all ingredients together and place in a spray bottle taking care to shake it well before using. This is a wonderful, lightly scented mist that you can use as you exercise or after a day of outdoor fun. Keep all unused portions in the refrigerator and no longer than a week.

Cleopatra's Milk Bath

2 Cups of dry milk powder

1/2 Cup cornstarch

5 drops of sandalwood essential oil

1/2 teaspoon of pure vanilla extract

one square piece of cheese cloth

Mix all ingredients in a small bowl until well incorporated. Place half the recipe in the middle of the cheesecloth square, forming a mound. Bring the four corners together and tie with a piece of string. Run a hot bath and place bag under running water. When bath has cooled to a comfortable temperature, gently squeeze the bag. At the end of the bath, quickly shower off any milk residue.

Shanghai Salts

2 Cups cornstarch

1 Cup rice flour

1/2 teaspoon ground cinnamon

1/4 Tablespoon ground dried ginger

1 Tablespoon cloves

10 drops essential orange oil

1/2-Cup Epsom salts

1 to 2 drops of yellow food coloring

Place all ingredients in a blender and mix well. Put 4 table-spoons in hot running water. Spicy and exotic, this is sure to become one of your favorite treats. Small candy jars with lids make the perfect containers. Store in a cool, dry place.

Crystal Salts

1/2 Cup of sea salt

1 Cup of baking soda

1/2-Cup Epsom salts

20 drops of lemongrass essential oil

A few drops of red food coloring (optional)

Mix all ingredients together until completely blended. Place in a pretty glass bottle using a natural seashell from the shore as a measuring scoop. Keep in a cool, dry place.

Love Bath

1 Cup freshly picked rose petals

1/2 Cup dried milk

10 drops rose essential oil

1 cheese cloth square

Combine all ingredients together in a bowl and transfer to the cheesecloth, forming a mound in the center. Bring the four corners together and tie with a piece of string. Run the bath water steaming hot and place bag under running water. When bath is at a comfortable temperature, take the bag and squeeze it a couple of times before entering.

Peppermint Candy Soak

2 Cups of spring or distilled water

1/2 Cup of loose peppermint tea or 2 tea bags

1/2-Cup Epsom salts

10 drops of peppermint essential oil

Bring water to a boil and add tea. Turn heat off and let steep for 1 or 2 hours depending on the strength you want. Remove tea bags and place all ingredients in a blender until incorporated. Clean glass bottles with corks or tops work best as containers. When ready to use, give the bottle a good shake and pour in as much as you desire to bath water. Store all unused portions in your refrigerator for no more than 2 weeks. Great for sore, tired feet as well. Very invigorating, so do not use it at night unless you are going dancing!

Mermaid's Lagoon

1 Cup of Epsom salts

1 Cup of coarse sea salt

10 drops frangipani fragrance oil or essential oil

10 drops of blue food coloring

Combine all ingredients well and place in a container with a lid. Epsom salts do have the tendency to evaporate. Light and refreshing, this will quickly become one of your favorite indulgences.

Star Burst

1 Cup of Epsom salts

1 Cup of baking soda

20 drops of strawberry fragrance oil

10 drops of yellow food coloring

1 vanilla bean, split open

Mix first four ingredients together in a large bowl. The reason this recipe calls for yellow food coloring instead of red to produce a pink color is because these salts are supposed to smell like delicious star fruit. Unfortunately star fruit scents are not easily accessible, therefore strawberry will suffice. Place the mixture in a clean container, putting the vanilla bean straight down the center. With time the vanilla bean will add a warm touch to your Star Burst salts. Let cure 2 weeks before using. Store in cool, dry place in a container with a tight fitting lid.

Queen of the Night Body Butter

8 Tablespoons jojoba or sweet almond oil (base)

1 teaspoon vitamin E

1 Tablespoon margarine

10 drops of jasmine essential oil

3 drops of vanilla essential oil

1/2 teaspoon of honey

1-teaspoon natural bees wax

Place all ingredients in a saucepan. Mix until completely melted and combined. Turn heat off and pour into a clean jar. Cover and place in the refrigerator. You may need to blend it a bit before using. A little goes a long way.

Complete Body Treatment

With this set of treatments you can turn your home into a lavish spa for a day. Be sure to look over all the steps first before proceeding and make adjustments to the concoctions depending on your skin type.

Almond Body Polisher

4 Tablespoons baking soda

1/2 Cup white corn meal

10 natural almonds

1 Tablespoon almond extract

In a coffee grinder place almonds and pulse until ground well. The same can be done in a blender. Blend all ingredients together and store in the refrigerator until ready to use.

Rose Water Clay Mask

1 Cup of rose Body Elixir

5 drops rose essential oil (optional)

Enough dry clay to make a thick mask

1 teaspoon sweet almond or olive oil

Stir together well and store in a clean container. Place in the refrigerator until ready to use.

Cherry Bath Oil

4 Tablespoons olive oil

2 Tablespoons canola oil

2 Tablespoons sweet almond oil

1/2 teaspoon vitamin E

10 drops of cherry fragrance oil

In a small bowl mix all ingredients together. Keep refrigerated until ready to use.

Violet Body Splash

2 Cups fresh violet flowers

3 Cups spring or distilled water

1/2 teaspoon vanilla extract

Heat water to a boil. Add flower petals and simmer for 15 minutes covered. Turn heat off and let sit 1 hour. Pour into a glass container or ceramic cup and keep refrigerated until ready to use. Strain off plant material and add vanilla extract. If fresh violets are not in season use one of the other Body Elixirs in this book.

Step one:

Wet skin before applying the Almond Body Scrub. Spread on Scrub and gently massage in a circular motion to remove dead skin. Rinse off with warm water.

Step two:

Apply Rose Water Clay Mask to arms, legs, thighs etc. keeping in mind to avoid sensitive skin areas. Spread on a thin layer and let dry for about 20 minutes.

Step three:

Draw a warm bath and add the Cherry Bath Oil. When water is a comfortable temperature enter and soak until clay can be wiped off easily with a wash cloth.

Step four:

Douse yourself quickly with the Violet Body Splash. If you like you can use the Queen of the Night Body Butter for an even more moisturizing effect.

Note: Remember to always do a patch test.

Facial formulas

Youth in a Bottle

10 drops rose essential oil

10 drops neroli essential oil

10 drops orange essential oil

1 Cup spring water

Place ingredients in order listed taking care to use a very clean glass bottle. Shake well before applying to freshly washed skin. Please do not substitute any of the essential oils for fragrance oils. The affect of this treatment will not be the same.

Rose Oil Rejuvenator

10 drops rose essential oil

2 Tablespoons sweet almond oil

3 drops geranium essential oil

Mix well. Keep in a glass bottle in the refrigerator. Use as spot treatment for wrinkles and/or fine lines or as an all-over face moisturizer. Do not use around the eyes.

Rose Facial Steam

1/2 Cup fresh rose petals or 1/4 Cup dried

5 drops rose essential oil (optional)

1/2 teaspoon vanilla extract

Enough water to fill a large bowl

Using a tea kettle bring water to a rolling boil. Place a large bowl on a hard, flat surface like a table. Add petals, extract and essential oil. Drape a bath towel over your head and pour water into the bowl. Move your face as close as possible to the steam without burning yourself. If steam is too hot, let it cool a bit. Stay under the towel for about 20 to 30 minutes. Use no more than once a week.

European Milk Cleanser

2 Cups dried milk

1 vanilla bean (optional)

5 drops of lavender

Mix together and place in a container with a lid. Store in a dark, cool place. To use, moisten a small amount in your hand with water and smooth over face and neck. Use the balls of your fingers to make small circular motions over your skin. Rinse well with warm water. Not only will this cleanse your skin but it will also help even-out your complexion.

Strawberry Yogurt Mask

1/4 Cup plain yogurt

3 fresh strawberries

3 drops of lavender essential oil

Remove the green leaves and stems from the strawberry. Using a fork smash it into a fine pulp. You can also use a blender or small food processor. Mix in yogurt and essential oil. Smooth over clean skin and leave on for 15 to 20 minutes. Wash off with warm water. You will find this mask quite soothing and cooling to the skin. Discard any unused portions.

Chapter 10

WHAT A MAN NEEDS
TO STAY YOUNG

■

Now if you men are thinking "A younger woman!" you too are barking up the wrong tree! I will say this. Studies have in fact shown that older men who have younger wives usually have healthier, longer lives. On the other hand, men usually fare worse after a divorce or death of their spouse, even though it is women who are most often worse-off financially as a single person. The truth is that marriage does a person good whatever your gender. Someone to share your dreams with, who validates your existence and contributions to the world, is a powerful charge to your life's force.

People in general do not fare well alone and some research has shown older people to have increased dementia and forgetfulness just from living on their own. Independence is important, I will not deny that. However, we have a need for human conversation and interaction throughout the day, every day. Men in particular have special needs in this area. One interesting poll showed that while women will list their sister or neighbor as their best friend, most of the men queried named their wives as their closest companion. So what does that tell you? Your relationship with your wife may be one of your best predictors of future health and well being. Jealousy, bitterness and power plays all diminish the value of a relationship and have no place in a happy marriage. Yet, we are all human and give in to these weaknesses from time to time. It is the constant "diet" of these negative feelings, however, that greatly increases your risk of strokes and heart attacks. The stress of a contentious relationship such as just described can undermine even the healthiest person's well being.

An added peril for men in this regard is that males are less likely to go get psychological help for problems such as depression and anxiety disorders. Society has taught men to not give into or express their feelings; that there is something weak in needed help for mental problems. So here you see a suicide rate in males that could be greatly reduced if these patients had reached out for the care they so desperately needed, but were afraid to ask for.

I am not saying that every time you feel a bit down because your favorite baseball team didn't get the pennant again this year is an indication for a trip to the psychiatrist. We are talking about depressive episodes that last more than two weeks and effect your quality of life. Such things as withdrawal from others, sudden loss of sex drive, hopelessness; lack of attention to personal hygiene and apathy about life are not normal. If you feel you have absolutely no reason for joy in living, you will need to stop and evaluate your circumstances. Far be it from me to give anyone advice on depressive disorders as I am not qualified to do so. However, I do know of the benefits of counseling my colleagues have to offer to people in this condition. Proper diet and even medication if needed may save your life. (Please read Chapter 13 on Middle Aged Blues).

A lot of things can be causing your problems. Ask yourself, have you recently been switched to a new medication? Are you getting enough sleep every night, at least 7 hours? Are you eating right and getting enough complex carbohydrates such as whole grains in your diet? This is information you will need to consult with your doctor. All the same, I personally would get a firm diagnosis from a physician trained in psychiatric disorders such as a psychiatrist. This is because a psychiatrist is a medical doctor who, over and above his medical training, has gone on to study the specific disorders of the mind. Your general practitioner might misdiagnose you and prescribe a less than effective therapy for your condition. Also a psychiatrist will be able to give you the full program support needed for the most complete recovery. It is not all about pills here. It is about getting down to what is actually at the root of your suppression or anxiety, if that is at all possible. That is not going to happen during your customary 15-minute office visit with your family doctor, either. Psychiatry is one field that requires patient participation to get better. People who require medication to treat their mental disorders, but are outpatients, often go off of their medications. This is because after a period of time, they decide that they are cured and no longer need the prescribed drugs. Taking medication also makes them feel as if they are ill, while not taking it makes them think that they are normal. It is at this point when most suicides, assaults and homicides take place involving this segment of the population. The accompanying use of street drugs, alcohol and lack of nutritious food add up to a powder keg ready to explode.

Therefore, your relationship's as they relate to your mental health and well being should not be taken lightly. It is much better to get these matters off your chest with someone, rather than let him or her fester into major issues. At the core of your self-care is nutrition. Realizing that these needs may change a bit as one gets older will allow you to prepare and supplement to offset some of these conditions.

TESTOSTERONE AND MALE MENOPAUSE

If you turn back to Chapter 2, you will see this article, but I am reprinting it here because most of you men will not bother to turn back to review it! The point is that just as estrogen production begins to wane for women during menopause, testosterone levels begin to drop in men as well with age. This causes changes in the size of the prostate. This is why experts recommend that men over age 40 get digital rectal exams as part of their yearly check up as well as PSA, (prostate specific antigen), assays. It is estimated that close to 28,500 men in the U.S. died of prostate cancer in 1989. This is actually a high mortality rate because this kind of cancer is about 90% treatable if caught early. Although its occurrence in men under age 50 is rare, if you are an African American male, you should note that your risk for developing prostate cancer is greatly increased over other races.

Not all types of male cancers occur with increased age either. Testicular cancer for example, is seen in younger men under age 30. This is why learning early examination techniques of the testicles is every bit as important as breast self-exam for women. Men with an undescending testicle are at an even a greater risk of developing testicular cancer. Consequently, for every man, here is the monthly drill:

Testicular Self Exam

Each testicle needs to be examined individually. Make sure you are in a warm place. Ideally the best time to do a testicular exam is after a warm bath when the scrotum is more relaxed. This is because heat causes the testes to move away from the body, as warmth immobilizes sperm. Hence, this is your body's way of maintaining sperm at the proper temperature for survival.

While standing up, place your thumbs on the front surface of the testicle while supporting it with the index and middle fingers of both hands. Now gently roll each testicle individually between the fingers and thumbs. Do you note any lumps, hardness or thickness especially when compared to the other testicle? What you may feel is the epididymis, which is a soft, tubelike body behind the testicle itself. This is normal. Also note that masses felt outside of the testicle are NOT tumors of the testes. So relax, you are done.

Whatever your age, a little self care goes a long way towards prevention. There is something else you will need to be vigilant about, and that is your exposure to toxic chemicals and heavy metals, specifically cadmium. Cadmium, (elemental symbol Cd) has the atomic weight of 112.40 and specific gravity of 8.65. Cadmium was discovered in 1817 by Friedrich Stromeyer and is a silver-white, lustrous, malleable, ductile metal. It is commonly used industrially in electroplating coatings on iron and steel to prevent corrosion and in atomic reactors.

When I worked for major industry, I was Quality Assurance Manager for an analytical chemist. Part of my duties were to coordinate the material safety data sheets for the company and teach Right to Know. Whatever company you work for, part of regulatory compliance is that you have complete access to these material safety data sheets and be taught how to protect yourself from hazardous chemicals stored on site. If you work in such a company, you need to familiarize yourself with the material safety data sheets or the MSDS's on cadmium. Data such as storage requirements, exposure levels and target organs effected by cadmium are included on its MSDS. They tell you the specifics about this metallic element, but this is something the information sheets will not tell you, so pay close attention here:

BPH AND THE CADMIUM CONNECTION
"Zinc and Selenium may be the Solution"

Benign Prostatic Hyperplasia, or BPH, has long been considered a wake up call, (often in the middle of the night), to the male physiological changes to be anticipated in mid-life. After about age 50, a man's testosterone decreases while other hormones such as prolactin and estradiol increase. Enlargement of the prostate occurs when testosterone entering the prostate cell is converted to dihydrotestosterone. It is this substance, DHT, which enters the cell nucleus and stimulates protein synthesis, which then causes the abnormal growth and enlargement of the prostate. The prostate will progressively crowd the urethra that passes through it. The effect is much like someone standing on a garden hose thus impeding the flow of water.

Damage to the kidneys and bladder infections are not uncommon to this condition. Primary symptoms include frequent trips to the bathroom and decreased urinary flow, which are evident in up to about 50% of all males by age sixty and close to 80% past age seventy. A total of close to 10 million American men are effected by this condition. Until recently, this was thought to be an inevitable part of the aging process. Now science has become aware of environmental and nutritional factors as playing a role in either helping or hindering this problem.

A controlled study showed that 14 out of 19 men exhibited improvement when they took the mineral zinc in the amount of 150 mgs daily for 2 months, with a maintenance dose of 50-100 mgs daily. This was demonstrated in 14 of the patients showing shrinkage of the prostate as assessed by rectal palpitation, X-ray and endoscopy. (Bush IM et al Zinc and the Prostate) Zinc is an essential mineral that is crucial to prostate gland function and the normal growth of reproductive organs. Deficiencies in zinc show up as hair loss, high cholesterol levels, impaired night vision, impotence, memory impairment and of course prostate trouble. The saddest part is that all of these symptoms are associated with just getting older!

Not to be overlooked are our modern day exposures to chemicals and heavy metals, many of which are carcinogenic or cancer causing. One observational study took a close look at cadmium exposure. Cadmium is a soft bluish-white metal used industrially is electroplating, batteries and atomic reactors. Prostatic cadmium concentrations in patients with BPH were measured by atomic absorption spectroscopy and were found to be considerably higher than in normal tissue, (23.11 +/- 3.28 vs. 5.25 = /- 0.62 nmol/g). Prostatic DHT levels were directly proportional to the cadmium concentrations.

There seems to be evidence that selenium, mentioned previously for cancer prevention, may protect cadmium-induced growth stimulation of the prostatic tissue or epithelium. Patients may undertake a non-invasive elemental analysis that can assess both toxic cadmium and beneficial selenium / zinc ratios. This is accomplished through a simple hair analysis.

So there you have it. An elemental hair analysis will not only indicate what you have been exposed to but what you may be lacking nutritionally, such as selenium and zinc levels. Men are generally good candidates for hair analysis as they tend to do less to their hair than us women, (i.e. coloring, perms, etc.) These chemical processes deposit chemicals on the shaft of the hair that may register as false positives for certain elements, specifically the sulfur and lead compounds. That is because both are used in permanent hair solutions and colorings. This is why hair should be clipped close to the scalp to get the best determination of elements present from an endogenous, (that coming from within), rather than an exogenous source.

Selenium is found in abundance in natural foods such as Brazil nuts, nutritional yeast, sea greens and seafood, (especially salmon), wheat germ and whole grains. Additionally there are many herbs that are rich in selenium as well. They include chamomile, hawthorn berry, milk thistle, nettle, raspberry leaf, rose hips and yellow dock. The benefits of hawthorn berry and raspberry leaf have already been highlighted in this book for the heart and regulation of female hormones respectively. This is why you only need to include a few herbs and supplements on your rejuvenating list. All of the nutritional adjuncts recommended in this book are designed to do double, even triple duty as they are so good for many "age" related disorders. You will find yourself saving quite a bit of money as a result and compliance will be easier as well.

Chapter 11

WHAT A MAN NEEDS
TO LOOK YOUNG

■

Once again a younger woman on your arm is not the answer I am thinking of for you! Due to the fact that women generally out-live men by an average of 5 years this sort of arrangement may leave a woman a very young widow. However, it does not necessarily have to be so. As previously mentioned in the last chapter, often times a younger partner for either sex can increase life satisfaction and lon-gevity in the older partner. We are not sure why but perhaps youthful optimism, willingness to try new things and the extra exercise one gets from having to keep up with a younger mate may be part of the answer. A younger woman may be more interested in keeping her older husband around by watching over his diet, preparing low fat, high fiber dishes and seeing that he keeps himself in shape. An older man, seeking to keep and please his younger wife may be more than willing to com-ply. Men, no matter what their age are naturally competitive. An older man knows that he needs to keep in shape to main-tain his edge in pleasing his young wife who may be attracted to younger men.

There is also evidence that having children, even late in life, has beneficial effects on either parent. Even grandparents who regularly care for grandchildren tend to be healthier and more mentally alert. Undoubtedly "youth rubs off"! Cosmetically we are seeing more men going in for plastic surgery to look younger and compete with more youthful peers for top positions. Men have an advantage over women in that their skin is thicker, therefore less prone to wrinkling. Also the act of shaving aggressively exfoliates the top layer of skin and encourages younger, fresher layers to emerge from below. Clean shaven men often appear more youthful as a result. Here is a natural shave lotion from *Secret Potions, Elixirs and Concoctions* published by Lotus Press, to enhance this process:

Ginger After Shave for Men

1/2 teaspoon fresh ginger

5 drops lavender

1/2 teaspoon honey

1 Cup water

Bring water to a boil. Reduce heat and add ginger. Simmer for 5 minutes and turn off heat. Let sit another 5 minutes. Strain off ginger and add essential oil and honey. Place in a glass bottle and refrigerate. This may be kept for up to a week and a half. Do not use if you have very sensitive skin.

Still, looking young is only part of the goal, for what good is repairing the facade when the understructure is failing? It is true that looking good helps your self esteem but if on the inside you feel like 120, a face lift is not going to do you all that much good. Our muscles begin to shrink as fat replaces them and that includes our facial muscles. Proper fat metabolism and muscle toning for the whole body is therefore very important.

Building Muscle Mass After Age 40

Actually there is no difference in your ability to build lean muscle tissue after forty than when you were 20! It is true that we lose 1% muscle per year after age 30, however people who are active will often offset this decline and retain their youthful physiques despite the advance of years. The real issue is that when we are younger, we are naturally more active. Rollerblading, swimming, hiking and bicycling are all activities associated with youth. Sometimes we are our own worse enemy in thinking that we are too old for these things or others would think so seeing us doing them. Perhaps we are not in the best of shape. Being self-conscious as to what others will think can likewise be a stumbling block to progress.

Joining a gym is for many a big commitment. Some people think, "Oh, I'll never go, it will be a waste of money." However when you see the monthly gym fees you will be paying, well that may very well motivate you to get yourself in gear! The first club I joined was for women only. I really liked it. A pool, Jacuzzi and sauna were some of the perks I enjoyed most. I took a few aerobics classes, used the body building equipment and got wonderful results. Then the boom lowered. They went out of business! I was one of the few fortunate ones who received their money back on what I had already paid for my remaining membership, but most did not. In limbo, I took private aerobic classes that were passable, but nowhere near as complete as the women's club. I later joined a Gold's Gym because it was on the way home from work. Since I had to pass it everyday, it was easy to schedule time to go. My day would start early and I would finish work at about 3pm and arrive at the gym around 3:45pm. I would work out on the machines for about 2 hours, maybe take a step class, shower, get into the sauna and dress to go home. The atmosphere there was that it was more like a social club with more men than women, all of whom seemed to be looking for dates. It is very distracting constantly saying, "No thanks," and I think I would have gotten more done in less time had I been in an all female environment.

So that is my experience. There are many options to choose from now as many gyms are seeing a drop off in new membership. The heyday of aerobics and healthy eating has diminished greatly from the 1980's through the mid-1990's. You want to know what is really hot now? Steakhouses! The pendulum has truly swung too far to the left. You may be able to get a better deal if you go in with a friend and join at the same time for a discount. Look for clubs that will assure that you have a personal walk-through of the facility and show you how to use everything. Gyms with pools, saunas and whirlpools may be a bit more expensive, but worth it as these are things that most of us do not have or wish to maintain at home. Choose according to what is important to you as well.

Gold's Gym is great for body building, aerobics and step classes. A New York Sports Club has similar programs including racquetball. Their layout may be more conducive to interacting with other club members in such competitive games. A woman's club such as Lucille Roberts and American Woman are more tailored to the needs of women. The training equipment is better proportioned to the female physique, with better padding, shorter bars, etc. Even when I did not have much of a chance to go that often, the years that I have belonged to a gym, any gym have been my very best for how I looked and felt. Even with my home unit, the Nordic Track Ultra Lift, I find that there is nothing like a club to motivate you and give you a little something special to look forward to on the weekends. Not that I will be tossing out my home exercise machine anytime soon, but it has its place as a complement to the club workouts, not replacing them.

If the gym has a personal trainer option, take it. This person can set up a program just for you, showing how to execute the exercise movements, lifts, etc. for maximum results and to avoid injury. You may only wish to enlist them for a very brief contract and then you are on your own, which is fine. Men do best with someone to spot them on the heavy equipment anyway so this is something to consider if you do not have a regular workout buddy. Make sure that you drink enough fluids before, during and after your workout and take a complete calcium supplement when you get home after your workout and just before bedtime. Why? Well, all of that muscle contraction has caused lactic acid and other metabolites of muscle activity to build up in your tissues. This is the ache you often feel in your muscles the next day. Getting enough absorbable calcium is therefore key to helping the muscle rid itself of impurities, including lactic acid, of which I previously spoke, which causes cramps and "Charlie Horses".

Another wonderful ally in pain relief is to have Arnica on hand. It comes in both a gel and a massage oil. The gel is most often used by football players. Arnica gel and ice are about all that is needed for a bad bruise. The Arnica gel alone helps control swelling, pain and bruising. The ice restricts blood vessels, keeping the blood flow to a minimum to the area of the contusion. It is almost miraculous how well this flower extract works. It is likewise just as good for sore, achy muscles. After your workout take a warm shower, and massage your aching, strained muscles with Arnica oil. The oil works slower than the Arnica gel so it will diffuse into the tissues over a longer period of time but give you more complete, longer lasting relief from muscle aches. The gel is almost like an immediate ice pack for pain of a bang or bruise. The Arnica oil soothes sore muscles thus making it an excellent massage oil for that application.

Armed with a health club that meets your specific needs and has the amenities you are looking for, you are now ready. Have the club assess your body fat percentage when you begin as well as take your measurements. Have a club representative show you how to use everything even if you are not particularly interested in using it at that time. Work with a trainer who will detail a program for you based on your own specific goals of building lean body mass. Be prepared by drinking enough fluids, getting adequate amounts of absorbable calcium and having plenty of Arnica on hand for after your workout. I guarantee, you will kiss the bottle!

To motivate you even further, people with a higher rate of lean muscle mass can eat more. This is because lean muscle tissue is always active, contracting, generating heat, thus expending energy. Adipose tissue, or fat, simply maintains itself by sitting there and accumulating. Your scale may not indicate much of a change but the way your body looks in your clothes and in the mirror will be much more toned, firmer and more compact. With a little time and a bit more effort you will have greater stamina, energy and poise. You will actually want to be active in other sports or events because your muscles are toned and coordinated. Not only will your muscles look good, they will perform better for you than when you were younger.

Note: You might wish to think of adding 2-3 grams of Calcium Pyruvate to your exercise protocol. It is excellent in helping your body to naturally turn carbohydrates into energy and putting on lean muscle mass as well.

Chapter 12

REGAINING YOUR MENTAL EDGE
Memory, Mental Acuity & Retention

■

"Dr. Miczak, I am starting to forget an awful lot. Could it be Alzheimer's?" I currently teach a course as adjunct faculty for Brookdale College in Lincroft, NJ. The name of the course is Super Memory with Nutrition and Herbs and it has never failed to draw top registration from the students. That is because everyone, young, old and otherwise wants to increase his or her mental edge and memory powers. We are also concerned about developing Alzheimer's, whose incidence increases with age. Most people have nothing to worry about, however if you have a parent with the disease, you may be at a greater risk than the general population.

It is thought that Alzheimer's carries with it a genetic link. However, there have been cases of identical twins who are genetically more alike than a parent and child. In these studies one twin who did not have the disease used anti-inflammatories on a regular basis, (i.e. ibuprofen, aspirin, etc.), while the other sibling did not. The results were that the healthy twin functioned at or above her age level in memory and mental acuity. The other had advanced Alzheimer's, was incontinent and required round the clock care including feeding. Keep in mind twins are obviously the same age. Thus the progression of the disease would have been the same for each twin if the link were purely genetic. *(Naturally occurring anti-inflammatories include the enzyme bromelain, which is derived from fresh pineapple and herbs of the mint family.)*

There is much we still need to learn about this disease. Rather than obsessing over if and when we will get it, our time might be better spent getting together as much data as possible to help ourselves as well as our loved ones who may be exhibiting similar symptoms. A confirmed diagnosis for Alzheimer's is still not available as of yet, outside of an autopsy where the destruction of brain cells can be clearly seen. There are specific eye drops that can be used where Alzheimer's patients will have a specific reaction, as a sign of a positive diagnosis. Still, even this test is not fool-proof and what if it is wrong? Do you want the mental burden of living under that sort of sentence, which may be inconclusive? I'm sure not. Take the initiative and read the following article. It will give you a better sense of empowerment as to what you can do now to save your memory.

GINGKO BILOBA'S EFFECT ON MEMORY

The use of Gingko Biloba in the treatment of age related disorders is still sparse and without much support from the medical community despite positive findings written in their own peer review publications such as *The Journal of the American Medical Association* (JAMA). Physicians often see individuals who subscribe to such alternative modalities as having a naive expectation of miracles even if in fact they would be pleased with modest improvements. The two conditions covered in this section both mention Alzheimer's and dementia, which are actually two different conditions. One can have senile dementia apart from Alzheimer's, as dementia can stem from other pathological processes.

Senile dementia is often the result of atherosclerosis or hardening of the arteries. These major arteries are responsible for providing adequate blood flow to the brain. These crucial arteries such as the cranial and carotid vessels can become partially or almost completely occluded with arterial "plaque," which prevents the artery from delivering the appropriate quantity of oxygenated blood to the brain. Victims of senile dementia will often hallucinate, thinking they are seeing visions or objects that are actually not there.

Alzheimer's is, on the other hand, due to an unknown etiology meaning it is not clear what causes the deterioration of brain tissue in these patients. The area that is attacked first is the area of the brain responsible for short-term memory. Old memories persist while more recent ones begin to slip with greater frequency. Doing simple math, remembering what day it is or the names of new acquaintances becomes increasingly more difficult. In embarrassment, many early sufferers begin to withdraw socially, which only makes matters worse.

Dementia may be present in the Alzheimer's patient as well, but different causes effect the same end; lack of normal blood profusion to brain cells. In the Alzheimer's patient as opposed to the senile dementia patient, the brain cells no longer exist to receive the necessary blood flow.

Alzheimer's is seen with increasing frequency proportionate to the patient's age although it can occur earlier in life. This type of early adult onset of the disease is suspect of being passed on by a recessive gene, as it has been seen to run in families. Current allopathic protocol recommends the use of Aricept or donepizil HCL. This drug will not cure the disease nor will it stop its progression. While it may not even help the patient at all, especially in the later stages, it is still prescribed because it can improve thinking ability in some patients. Not exactly great odds for improvement and none for the arrest of the disease. Also worthy of consideration is the fact that Aricept has associated side effects and risks such as commonly documented diarrhea, muscle cramps, nausea and insomnia. Why aren't comparatively safer products such as Gingko being explored and studied, since it holds out no more or less hope than these existing prescription therapies?

We have to assume that at least three issues come into play here that would explain this.

1. There is not much money being funneled into research for this segment of the population's specific health concerns.

2. There is a pervasive attitude that this is the normal course of aging and there is something wishful, perhaps even unnatural, about trying to alter its course.

3. Ginkgo is an herb. As an herb it is a product of public domain and cannot be patented by any one pharmaceutical company or entity.

That withstanding, here is an excerpt from an informative article that describes the research showing the preliminary indication that Gingko may be of help to Alzheimer's patients:

SCIENCE NEWS UPDATE
Gingko Biloba Can Stabilize and Even Improve Dementia
Changes substantial enough to be noticed by caregivers

WASHINGTON, D.C. - "An extract of Ginkgo Biloba can stabilize and in some cases improve the cognitive functions and the social behavior of demented patients for six months to one year according to an article in the October 22, 1997 issue of *The Journal of the American Medical Association's* (JAMA) theme issue on aging."

A doctor LeBars from the New York Institute for Medical Research in Tarytown, NY has studied and reported on the beneficial effects of EGb 761, which is a potent extract of Gingko Biloba. Their study used 309 demented patients with mild to moderately severe mental impairment caused by Alzheimer's, vascular dementia or a combination of both.

It was at the American Medical Association's 16th Annual Science Reporters Conference that LeBars presented his findings. His were the first empirical clinical trials using Gingko Biloba extract to be conducted in the United States. The clinical trial spanned one year and was a double blind, (neither the researchers nor the participants knew placebo from active compound), placebo controlled, parallel-group, multicenter study. In other words, every precaution was taken to assure that the results would be totally objective and representative of the herbal extracts efficacy or actions.

LeBars and his fellow researchers concluded: "EGb appears to stabilize and in an additional 20% of cases, (vs. placebo), improve the patient's functioning for periods of six months to one year. Regarding its safety, adverse side effects associated with EGb were no different from those associated with placebo."

The researchers found that 27 percent of patients treated 26 weeks or more with EGb achieved at least a four-point improvement on the 70 point Alzheimer Disease Assessment Scale-Cognitive subscale, (ADAD-Cog is the name of the scale), as compared with 14% on placebo. On another scale called the Geriatric Evaluation by Relative Rating Instrument of (GERRI), 37% had improved in their daily living and social behavioral skills as compared to 23% on placebo.

40% on placebo actually got worse while 23% improved so we can glean from these figures the relative effectiveness of Gingko Biloba extract.

The extract used in these clinical trials is very popular in Europe and is more concentrated than the Gingko Biloba herb capsules made from the whole plant. EGb, or extract of Ginkgo, has recently been approved in

Germany for the treatment of dementia even though how this herb works on the brain is not completely understood. Gingko does contain compounds that scavenge free radicals, which are thought to be the mediators of excessive brain fat oxidation and cell damage seen in the central nervous system of Alzheimer's patients.

The primary facts shown by this study is that EGb had a determinable effect on patients who were cognitively impaired, (having difficulty with normal thought processes). It also showed improvements in the daily living and social behavior of patients diagnosed with dementia. Caregivers were perhaps the main group to note these improvements as a result of their day to day interaction with these patients.

Researchers state: "Compared with the placebo group, the EGb group included twice as many patients whose cognitive performance improved and had as many whose social functioning worsened. In clinical terms, improvement on the ADAS-Cog scale of four points may be equivalent to a six month delay in the progression of the disease." (Read the complete article in JAMA 1997; 278:1327-1332)

Gingko's forte is in helping to improve circulation and oxygen transport to the brain. It also helps combat age-related memory loss, slow mental processing, dizziness, tinitus or ringing in the ears and even depression. Not only Alzheimer's patients stand to benefit either. Studies have shown improvement for Parkinson's sufferers as well.

It is worthy of note that support for this study was provided by Willmar Schwabe Pharmaceuticals. This would be rare for an American Pharmaceutical company to undertake because, as previously mentioned, they cannot patent an herbal product. Since it costs some 400 million dollars to bring a new drug from drawing board through market, they will not likely research a compound that they cannot hold rights to.

This study was enough proof for Warner Lambert who is now marketing EGb 761 extract as was used in this study under the line of herbal supplements called Quanterra. Warner Lambert is a pharmaceutical drug manufacturing giant with headquarters in Morristown, New Jersey. It is therefore quite radical of them to market an herb, namely Gingko Biloba. They have a patented, standardized extract of 24% flavone glycosides and 6% terpene lactones in the finished product, although this is also available from non-pharmaceutical herb manufacturers.

Although they point to the same clinical research as herb manufacturers do, many doctors and pharmacists that are familiar with the Warner-Lambert name will more than likely recommend their Gingko over others. You will see their ads in some consumer magazines because this product is marketed OTC, or over the counter. However, the greatest emphasis in advertising is made in trade and peer reviewed journals such as US Pharmacist. The ad for Quanta EGb 761 touts: "Supported by more well-controlled clinical studies than any other Gingko Biloba extract." They go on to say that it is supported by 7 placebo-controlled clinical trials and is clinically proven effective and well tolerated. Well, sorry to burst your bubble but EGb 761 is not a proprietary compound. In other words, any company, including herb manufacturers can manufacture this extract!

Still the Quanterra line with all of its pharmaceutical trappings must still have the requisite asterisk with the disclaimer that "These statements have not been evaluated by the FDA."

It also cannot patent the herb even though the process of standardization changes their product into a more concentrated extract containing those specific plant constituents. All the same it may just be smoke in mirrors. Gingko remains a product of public domain and will remain so unless the pharmaceutical companies are able to demonstrate alteration of the essential molecules, creating a new compound totally un-like that which is found in nature.

Perhaps the best advice in choosing a Gingko herbal product is to use an extract similar to what was used in the clinical trials here stated. There is a lot of controversy about this. Many traditional herbalists oppose using standardized products. They do have a point in saying there are compounds inherent to the whole herb and it is perhaps best not to "fool with Mother Nature". Actually, that is not what standardization is all about. Remember I worked for an analytical chemist. Before becoming Quality Assurance Manager, I ran chemical assays on batches of products for manufacturers. We used sophisticated photospectometry instruments that would read the chemicals present in a compound like a lie detector, for lack of a better analogy. This means that when placed in the machine for a chemical assay, we had a control sheet of what the compound should look like. Every time the instrument detected the requisite chemical compound it would register a peak or a valley on the scaled paper printout. After the photospectometry was complete, we would match the compound's print-out to that of our control or "model" sheet. If they matched, you had a good batch. This same instrumentation is used in every FDA approved pharmaceutical manufacturer, and our laboratory was no exception.

Likewise is the case with standardization. The whole herb is still used, but the final product or extract is checked to make sure the "active" ingredients are present. Now I am not going to open a debate on the importance of the isolated active compounds, (i.e. glycosides, flavanoids), over the other constituents present in the product but I will say this. Factors such as where and how the plant is grown, rainfall, soil conditions and even how the plant is stored after harvesting will play a part in that herb's potency from harvest to harvest, batch to batch. The only thing standardization does is assure you of the same amount or presence of those specific compounds with each run. It is that simple.

Extracts of Gingko Biloba are used in Germany and in the previously cited American study because the patient would have to take much more of the whole herb to achieve that same effect, if at all. Compliance is always a problem, so if you can find a concentrated Gingko extract that is time - released, you may be able to get away with once a day dosing. Keep in mind, however that the recommended daily dosage of Gingko Biloba extract to improve your brain function is between 120-160 mgs. You cannot expect immediate results either as Gingko takes about six months to take effect, or longer, if you are using the whole herb. Hence the more immediate results may be seen from taking the more concentrated Gingko Biloba extract instead. This is because standardized extracts are made from the dried leaves and contain a higher concentration of the active ingredients than, let's say, a tea made from the Gingko leaves. Follow the amount to take as suggested on the label by the manufacturer or take 40mgs of the extract three times daily for a total of 120 mgs. Also remember to take your Gingko extract before meals for maximum absorption.

AMPAKINES TO REJUVENATE SHORT TERM MEMORY

22 years ago in Hungary, the country of origin of my family surname, scientists discovered a treatment for senility and disorders involving blood flow to the brain. The class of drugs they discovered were ampkines. Today such medications that have been shown to enhance brain function are easy to get in Europe, with doctors widely prescribing them. This class of drugs are well tolerated and when tested on humans have shown no side effects. Even so ampakines have made their way to the U.S. but lack FDA approval because they are classified as nutritional supplements.

One such ampakine product that has come to us from Europe is vinpocetine. It is derived from an extract of the periwinkle plant, which is a spreading evergreen subshrub with purplish-blue flowers that bloom from spring throughout the summer. Researchers have isolated an alkaloid, vincamine, in the periwinkle, which benefits cerebral blood flow. Now the FDA has approved vinpocetine as a dietary supplement in the allowed amounts of 5 milligrams per tablet. It is not terribly expensive, either, which is a relief from the price gouging often seen in prescription drug products.

Vinpocetine is helpful in enhancing blood flow to the brain, thus facilitating oxygen utilization. There are even more recent studies that show it provides direct protection against the decline in the central nervous system's function due to the effects of aging. Vinpocetine actually works in a similar fashion as the popular drug, Viagra. Both work by increasing blood flow, but vinpocetine's action is specific to supplying tissues of the brain only. Therefore this "smart drug" has both protective and corrective properties that can help individuals before symptoms of senility even begin to appear. However, whatever your status, vinpocetine can improve blood flow to the brain, increasing oxygen utilization and thought processes.

Chapter 13

FIGHTING THE MIDDLE-AGED BLUES

■

Often times we will feel down as a result of circumstances and also for no discernible reason. Our hormones, brain chemistry and energy levels all play a role in how we will feel from day to day.

IS WINTER MAKING YOU SAD?
SEASONAL AFFECTIVE DISORDER
By Dr. Marie Miczak

The American Psychiatric Assoc. includes Seasonal Affective Disorder, (SAD), also called the "winter blues," as a distinct subcategory of affective disorders. Although there are many variations, this type occurs as the days begin to shorten in the fall and continues until spring returns. Typical symptoms include many of the same complaints observed in depression; sadness, decreased libido, withdrawal from social activity and impaired general functioning. To make matters worse there is also an excessive need for sleep, marked daytime fatigue, increased appetite and cravings for sweets with its resultant weight gain.

In an effort to combat this disorder, a number of prescription medications and psychotherapies are used, often with
measurable success. However many antidepressant medications also have adverse side effects. As an alternative phototherapy, or the use of light boxes, is safe and often quite effective as well. Such units are used extensively in Alaska where
this condition is seen most frequently. Along with light therapy
as described below, there are simple things anyone can do to
improve your mood year round:

1. Lighten up! Many SAD patients begin phototherapy with a
   20-minute length of exposure first thing in the morning. Try
   taking a brisk walk in the early morning daylight. The light
   exposure combined with the aerobic exercise supplied by
   walking releases endorphins or our body's own "feel good"
   chemicals.

2. Hypericum perforatum or Saint John's Wort. Researchers
   have uncovered components in this herb that effect brain
   chemistry to the improvement of one's mood and mental
   outlook. Note: Do not use if taking a medication in the
   category of a selective serotonin reuptake inhibitor or (SSRI)
   such as Zoloft, Prozac or Paxil.

3. Scent your world. Distinct essential oils stimulate the neurological centers of the brain to increase relaxation and a
   sense of well being. Popular plant essences for this purpose
   include rose, orange, lavender, jasmine and ylang ylang.
   Five drops of any of these in a full bathtub diffuses the es-
   sence into the air for an uplifted mood and better quality
   sleep.

4. Food for your mood. Your craving for starches and sweets
   may be your body's way of signaling a dip in serotonin. This
   neurotransmitter is important in controlling depression as
   well as compulsive behavior such as routine food bingeing.
   To help the body produce its own serotonin, include complex carbohydrates supplied by whole foods such as brown
   rice and potatoes.

If you feel that you have any type of mental disorder, it is important to seek professional diagnosis and treatment. For a psychiatrist referral in your area contact Marcia Bennett of the American Psychiatric Assoc. at (202) 682-6325 or e-mail mbennett@psych.org. In any event there is much that can be done to stave off the "winter blues" safely and naturally.

Part of the problem often times related to depression is that of stress. Young or old we all have it but too much can age you far beyond your years. A good example is to look at a president of the United States on his inauguration day. Hopeful, full of promise, even youthful. Now fast forward to the end of his 4-year term. Sometimes you can hardly recognize him! This is because the stress of being commander in chief, scrutinized in the public eye and responsible for the future of millions of people is very stressing and aging. Stress can sap the youthful vigor out of almost anyone's step. Even more it can lead to the onset of many diseases associated with modern life and even cause loss of memory and mental acuity as seen in my syndicated newspaper article below:

SECRETS TO SHARPENING YOUR MEMORY & THOUGHT PROCESS

Stress can truly be called the new disease of our modern world. Not that our ancestors didn't have stress, because they did. However as our world becomes smaller due to globalization of information, we have stimulus coming in from every corner of the world. Problems that our ancestors never dreamed about are now delivered to our doorstep each and every morning or even more frequently if you have Internet access.

All of this strains the human psyche beyond the limits of tolerability. It has often been said that technology often runs ahead of the abilities of its users. This is very true. For example ten years ago, I had to learn how to use an average of 10 different computer applications and programs per year. Today, this is my monthly average and I have to do it faster than

I did in the past. Upgrades, downloads, reinstallation's, reconfigurations, submissions on and on. I am responsible for maintaining all of my computerized equipment including everything from my P.C.'s to lab analyzers or I don't work! Everything is computerized.

This is great for the brain but because these applications are linked to my livelihood, it carries with it extra pressures to do it right and keep up. Since I am an admitted technology buff, I insist on having the latest gadgets and devices as well, which does not make matters any easier.

So the point is that due to the need to make a living, many of us are under similar pressures at work. Downsizing means fewer employees to share the office workload. Added duties with no pay increase to show for it is very daunting even for the most dedicated of workers.

Remember that stress also depletes the brain of serotonin, which is already seen as lacking in depressed patients. Serotonin is an important neurotransmitter responsible for maintaining a positive mood. Other important brain chemicals are likewise depleted during the triggered fight or flight responses. This has been associated with the inability to remember things under stress. Temporary loss of memory function is therefore linked to stress. This is why keeping up with deadlines is so important. When you are pressed at the last minute to complete a project, both you and the task suffers. You may not remember everything you wanted to include while under such pressure. Avoidable mistakes also tend to rear their ugly heads on projects with a quickly nearing deadline.

Part of the problem is lack of organization. I have used a Sharp Wizard electronic organizer since my lab days when I worked for an analytical chemist. Addresses, phone numbers, appointments and memos go with me wherever I go. Each day I have a "to-do" list that carries over if it is not completed. I am also able to schedule such items weeks or even months ahead of time, giving me the opportunity to prepare. The very act of writing down your appointments and memos also helps assist in memorizing what you need to do from day to day. Seeing it in your appointment book is another reaffirmation of the information and will help you remember it.

Keeping your mental edge under such pressures of daily life is not a simple task as I have just described above. However there are some excellent ways to keep yourself sharp and even improve your memory. Here are some suggestions taken right from my Brookdale college course, Super Memory with Nutrition and Herbs:

- If you are trying to learn new information very quickly, try sleep teaching. Get a pillow speaker at your local Radio Shack or electronics store. Place an audiotape of whatever you want to learn in a tape player hooked up to the pillow speaker which, as the name implies, is placed under your pillow. Turn on the tape and listen as you fall off to sleep. Using this method, you can learn any subject that is taught and recorded on the tape. Any language, book, subject, even a speech you need to memorize...anything! Play the tape every night for at least a month for maximum effect and see how much you will know.

- Focus. Most of us when presented with a new acquaintance do not remember the person's name because we were distracted when we were first introduced. Block all of that out and concentrate on the person's name. It also helps if you associate the person with a humorous idea. If the person's name is Gail Kolinsky simply remember a "girl" for Gail throwing a piece of coal into the sky, (coal in-sky = Kolinsky). Even if you do not recall Gail's first name, at the very least you will retrieve the mental image of her pitching a lump of coal into the sky. This is no problem because at the very least you will say, "Hello Ms. Kolinsky". Flattered that you even remembered her last name she will most likely say, "Oh please, do call me Gail!"

- To memorize lists of objects simply connect them in a humorous story. Let's say you want to go to the market. Skip the list and try this instead. You know you need carrots, garbage bags, apples and chicken breasts. Simply imagine the chicken breasts as a super hero action figure! The breasts have carrots for legs, an apple for the head and the garbage bag is its cape. Sounds odd? Who really cares? It is your own private system and who is to know? You can make up similar connections for multiple items on a list by adding a story line. The crazier the better because you WILL remember it. Try it. I guarantee that you will not only remember everything on your list, but you will have a good laugh everytime you go shopping as well.

- Do something pleasurable each day or when you are overwhelmed with work. This is often truly difficult because when you are behind, you are thinking, "I've got to get this done!" and press yourself beyond the limits of your mental output for the time. This is really when downtime is needed. Try taking a 15-minute vacation by taking a warm bath with a little rosemary and lavender essential oil in the bath water. These essential oils are the aromatherapeutic rescue aid that you need for both mind and body. The warm water helps the brain release endorphins or feel-good chemicals related to relaxation and well being. The rosemary reignites both your mental acuity and memory while the lavender helps you to de-stress. Peppermint also has this quality of reinvigorating the mind and body. Experiment with combinations of these for your own special super aroma blend.

Now you can continue driving yourself beyond all limits and end up with poor health and an inability to think and be creative therefore producing substandard or at best mediocre work. To me this does not sound like much of an option. You will end up having to do the work over again anyway due to too many mistakes, so what is 15 minutes? We are often our own worse enemy in this regard. If you belong to a health club, which I highly recommend, schedule some time just for you there. The change of scenery, activities, classes, pool, whatever is your fancy will help you to become much more productive. Stress, depression and exhaustion are all intense energy-zappers. You can work yourself to death, not so much from the activity but from not maintaining your personal health along the way. Everything about and for us gets placed on the back burner, especially for us women. Keep in mind, though, that you cannot continue to effectively care for everyone's needs while neglecting your own for very long without suffering the consequences. The problem is that your loved ones suffer with you when you are so depleted of anything else to give that you now need to be taken care of! That is a very sad statement indeed. I am not advocating narcissism here. However there has to be balance in our daily lives.

Trying to be "Super Mom or Super Woman" is futile. At some point along the way you are going to have to enlist reinforcements. Society is not going to give you any assistance in asserting yourself in this regard either. Just look at everyday commercials. A child deliberately makes a stinking mess, (sorry, that's me British blood starting to boil), and immediately appears super mom or actually super maid to clean it up. The child isn't even reprimanded and happily the mother proceeds to scrub and clean little Billy's crayon, marker and food splatters. Oh please, do give me a break. What does this teach the child about women and the value of your time? That is right, that mommies are supposed to do this, (see if they ever try this when the "old man" is watching them), and that your time is not really that important. These same children, especially male children, grow up with this sexist view that is carried over into the corporate world, firmly establishing the glass ceiling many women are trapped by. Likewise in the home environment, they are reluctant to help their wives around the house because they have been taught that a woman's true purpose is to serve them to the exclusion of other pursuits of importance to her.

So unless we start letting others know that taking care of ourselves is just as important as caring for the whims of everyone else, we will continue to be treated accordingly. Accustomed to this sort of coddling, your family may not want to let a good thing go. Guilt trips, whining and petty complaining are often ways to get you to do what they want, not what you need to do. Who then pays the ultimate price? The entire family, because at some point you will have nothing more to give. Burned out, confused and depressed, you will have nothing to offer your family but misery in seeing you in that condition. You will look and feel decades old before your time. If you get nothing else of value from this book, take home this one point. Invest in your own personal care on a daily basis and make it a priority. Your physical and mental health depend on it.

Chapter 14

THE MIND-BODY-SPIRIT CONNECTION TO STAYING YOUNG

■

Often overlooked is the intrinsic connection between youthfulness and spiritual well being. It is a known fact that individuals who engage in youthful activities are more apt to remain fit both physically and mentally. We only need look at individuals who are deprived of social and physical interaction to see the damaging effects. This can come at any age but is more pronounced in the elderly that have lost a mate and many lifelong friends over time. Case in point. Often when one spouse dies, it is quite common to see the other follow even though they may not have had any pre-existing medical conditions. Could this perhaps be what is considered dying of a broken heart?

This phenomenon even transposes itself into our relationships with the animal world. Did you know that owning a pet can lower your blood pressure? Yes, the act of petting your dog or stroking your cat actually begins the process of relaxation and decreases your blood pressure to more normal levels. It is also found that people who have pets invariably live longer as well. Perhaps it is knowing that another being relies on you for care and attention that perpetuates the life force in us all. We're not sure of the mechanics but this has been seen to be the case. If we look to one of the greatest literary works ever composed, the Bible, we see that Adam and Eve freely communicated and cared for the animals in their garden paradise. The Bible even says that the animals came to Adam to be named by him according to their specific attributes. Adam spent time observing the animals and their habits before naming them as he was charged with both their care as well as stewardship over their garden home. This is a highly charged spiritual plane that man was meant to exist in. We are here to care for, not dominate, the animals. We are here to cherish and cultivate the earth, not destroy it. When our lives fall out of harmony with these primal objectives, we suffer the effects of not being in step with the floor plan of the universe.

We may not have all the answers as to why these relationships with both our human and animal earth dwellers are so important to our longevity. However, we do know that people who spend time with others in a social atmosphere suffer less stress and anxiety. The very act of laughing is the best cardiovascular exercise imaginable! Likewise the simple act of telling a friend your troubles has an unburdening effect on your psyche. How often have you been close to tears over what seemed to be an insurmountable problem only to find yourself laughing about the ordeal after speaking with a close companion? This is because when left to our own devices, we often imagine an issue to be of earth shattering magnitude when it is not. However, after speaking with someone who has endured the same set of circumstances or perhaps worse, we too begin to see matters more positively. This is why the companionship factor is so important in the mind - body connection in maintaining a youthful persona.

Loneliness is indeed a silent killer as many seniors have found. That is why there is an increase in community volunteers from this segment of the population. Seniors are finding happiness and fulfillment by donating their time to help others who are less fortunate than themselves. This hearkens back to the benefit many people derive from caring for someone or something else such as a pet. Looking outside of our own needs and concerns while reaching out to help others may offer a benefit which to date is incalculable. Man has built within him a truly altruistic spirit. This is the motivating factor that causes a person to enter a burning building and save a stranger. Fear and concern over personal injury and peril are for a moment set-aside as the individual responds to another human's need for help. Enforcing this is the Bible's admonition where Jesus is quoted as saying, "No greater love has a man that he would lay down his life in behalf of his friend." This is an inherent human need to love and extend oneself in the service of others. In this we find the greatest joy in giving.

When we view the medical profession's ability to evoke a healing or to condemn one to a premature death, we then look at the mind-body connection and the power of suggestion. It is a well-known fact that when a person has faith in their health care provider, patient outcomes are often optimal. A positive bedside manner, cheerful concern and warm involvement in the patient's well-being are all earmarks of a top medical professional. On the other hand, a physician who follows a negative outlook with pessimism as his stock in trade steals hope from the very bosom of each of his patients. This is what is known as the "nocebo" effect. This is when you go to a doctor and receive a negative prognosis. Rather than offer you any hope whatsoever or even investigation of alternative therapy, your doctor says you will be dead in six months. Now depending on how much faith you have in that doctor's word, his death sentence may indeed become a reality for you. So rather than benefit from a placebo effect which is calculable in any and every double blind study, you will experience a "nocebo" or negative placebo effect. This sort of thing can be devastating to a patient who was already on the verge of emotional collapse due to fear and anxiety over their illness. Hence what the mind perceives the body fulfills. This can be readily seen in patients who have been misdiagnosed with a terminal illness and expire according to the doctor's prognosis despite the mistake. We don't know if it is the person's giving up on the pursuit of life or if such negative news has left them stripped of the will to live. Perhaps it is a combination of both with the added factor of simply giving in to what the doctor has prescribed as the inevitable.

While we don't yet have all the answers, empirical wisdom has proven time and time again that a person's mental and spiritual outlook are key factors in maintaining health. Youthful individuals are interested in their environment and others with whom they share it. This is achievable despite advanced age, as curiosity is a clear trait of an active, flexible mind needing to be filled with new experiences and sensations. The quest for knowledge need not cease as we age. In fact, we are finding more and more senior citizens returning to school to obtain degrees which perhaps they may never use secularly. Such individuals have seen the value of education extend far beyond the ability to earn a paycheck. They see their newly obtained degree as a sign of accomplishment and achievement despite their advanced age. That in and of itself is a very validating factor that they are still viable contributors to human society whether or not they choose to utilize their diploma in the work place. As humans, we all need this same sort of validation. That is a reason to remain among the living and vital throng of mankind rather than sit idle while the world passes by.

We can see how many have lost their youthful vigor and interest in life due to negative experiences, which they have allowed to overwhelm them. Notice I say, "they have allowed". We often put our own happiness in the hands of others. When a relationship fails, when our parents disappoint us, when we didn't get the support we felt we needed, are all issues that many people rely upon to explain their present state. This is not to say that traumatic experiences in one's childhood and even adulthood do not contribute to emotional distress and mental illness. However, in the toss and turbulence of human existence we all experience peaks and valleys, hope and tragedy, triumph and disappointment. If we assign our lack of success as human beings to the acts or even in-actions of others, then we are forever subject and dependent on outside sources for joy. This even extends to individuals who become dependent on drugs and alcohol to cope with their feelings of disappointment and unhappiness. Once again the assignment is given to someone or something else as being the source of completeness in one's life. Often lessons showing this to be a self-destructive thought process are learned too late.

When you become a parent you find out that your parents really did the best job they knew how to do. When you are involved in a relationship you find out how difficult it is to always be supportive of your partner. Likewise it often is not until you are much older that you realize that the things that you obsessed over as being so horrible in your youth are really of no magnitude at all in comparison to what you have seen in your lifetime. This is why when you told your parents about being humiliated in school by your classmates, time and experience have already taught them that this is no big issue and more serious problems await you further down the road. Now for that, many young people feel that their parents don't understand them. However they are just looking at a wider field of experience and comparing their child's problems to the greater ones seen later on in life. At best, a perception problem but this in no way means that the parent does not care for or support the child. On the other hand parents have to realize that children do not automatically draw conclusions as to love and acceptance based on obvious actions. Parents know from experience that feeding, clothing and housing a child denotes acceptance of responsibility and commitment to that child's well-being. Yet a child may not see it quite that way due to lack of experience in life. In keeping with the child's perceptions, a parent may need to demonstrate much more overt displays of affection and attention to assure that these needs are being met. It is not enough to assume that the child should know of the parent's love based on actions of parental responsibility.

It is never too late for the spirit to be nurtured. It is never too late for the spirit to be renewed, for such is the condition of the human heart which allows it to forgive, forget and be reborn with new hope. There's a saying that hope springs eternal from the heart of a fool. This really should read that hope springs eternal from the heart of the youthful. It is that optimism and belief in all possibilities that keeps us young. Likewise it is the distrust and jaded perception in life that ages us far beyond our chronological years. When we lose hope we wither and die from within despite the fact that we still live and breathe. In this way, the spirit has its last whim with us. Once broken it is so difficult to repair. Once lost it is so difficult to regain, but such is the substance of human existence. Our life force depends on it just as much as it depends on love and affection to tend the emotions.

One final example of the importance between the spirit, the mind and the body is an experience from Victorian times. During the 1800's it was common practice that children should be seen and not heard. Most often allowing a child to cry unattended was thought to be a step in building character in the infant. Nowhere were the disastrous effects of this type of doctrine seen more than in the orphanages of the time. According to strict medical practice of the day, nurses were told not to handle the infants any more than necessary; that would be only to feed and change the child. Other types of holding or interaction were thought to spoil the child or even expose it to disease. These hospitals adopted the sterile approach that lasted until modern-day maternity wards where mothers are often not encouraged to not hold their babies until it is time to take them home. During these dark days of the 19th century, due to these cold clinical practices in the handling of infants, mortality rates soared. Babies were dying in droves in these orphanages despite being well fed and clothed. What then was causing the higher rates of death? We later found that children lacking human touch simply withered away. Babies need to be held. Babies need to be touched. Above and beyond providing for their obvious needs, these emotional needs are integral to their survival. Change did come albeit slowly. The more progressive orphanages began to place rocking chairs in the nursery area and to assign more nurses to devote additional time to nurture and hold the babies. The result? Infant mortality dropped dramatically! Nothing had changed as far as their feeding and clothing. The only difference now was that the babies were receiving much more one on one attention from the nurses. This was enough to stem the tide of failing to thrive for these infants.

Hence we can learn a valuable lesson that there is indeed a need to be loved and cared for regardless of our age or position in life. It all boils down to preserving the fragile human spirit within us all. Without it our youthful zest for life cannot survive.

COMPANY RESOURCES FOR EXERCISE EQUIPMENT

■

FAMILY HEALTH AND FITNESS EQUIPMENT

Bicycles

MBC Discount Bikes
"Your Discount Family Fitness Center"
868 Main Street
Belford, NJ 07718 (Belford section of Middletown)
Store: (732) 471-1511

- Sales, expert repairs and service. Custom fitting for bicycles to suit your size and shape.
- Mountain, beach, exercise bikes and custom accessories for the entire family.
- Shipping available for most items to anywhere in the U.S.!

Visit On-line for trails, biking clubs and tips:
www.mbc.genxer.net

Rebounders

Needak Softbounce Mini-Trampoline
Visit On-line at: www.needak-rebounders.com
or call: (800) 232-5762

Needak hosts an educational website on the sport of rebounding and provides an airtight warranty on their products, which are manufactured in America. One of their top units is their 1/2 folding mini trampoline that folds to resemble a taco and comes with its own carrying case.

Being completely portable, you can take your unit outside, to the beach on vacation, etc. Retailing for around $240.00, it is a real bargain as you will get years of joint sparing aerobic exercise from it.

INDEX

ABOUT THE AUTHOR

■

Marie Miczak, D.Sc., Ph.D. is an alumni of Rutgers University College of Pharmacy where she is to this day an active member of the alumni association. Dr. Miczak holds a doctorate in Nutrition Science and is certified with the American Association of Nutritional Consultants. She also holds a doctorate in a branch of Pharmacognosy, (the study of medicines derived from plants and natural sources), and is a member of the American College of Clinical Pharmacology and the American Pharmaceutical Association's Academy of Science and Research.

Dr. Miczak is adjunct professor for Brookdale and Clayton Colleges as well as a visiting professor for universities across the nation. She is a frequent guest on network television appearing as an expert in her field of nutraceuticals on both TV and radio. Her syndicated columns are published and read internationally and she is a prolific author of over 4 books.

Dr. Miczak has a whole series of books dedicated to protecting your health with little known facts about adverse interactions and alternative medicine detailing both the benefits and the risks. The name of the series is *How Not to Kill Yourself* and is published by Random House. The first title in this series is *How Not to Kill Yourself with Deadly Interactions...When Herbs, Drugs, Foods and Vitamins Don't Mix*. For more information about Dr. Miczak's courses or how to order her books visit her website: www.miczak.com

To schedule a speaking engagement, interview or media appearance call toll free, 1-877-234-5350, ext. 676.

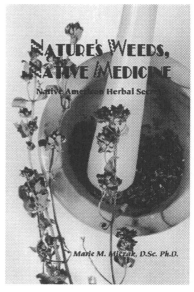

Back to Eden
Revised & Updated Edition

by Jethro Kloss

If you are interested in simple and effective alternatives to today's expensive and impersonal high technology, try this classic and comprehensive guide for safe and inexpensive natural remedies for the prevention of disease and sickness.

In Jethro Kloss's words, "God has provided a remedy for every disease that may afflict us. If our scientists would put forth the same efforts to find the 'true remedies' of nature that they do in the manipulation of chemicals, we would soon find the use of poisonous drugs and chemicals eliminated and sickness would be rare indeed."

Over **5 million** copies sold and still selling strong. This book is one of those rare phenomena which are truly epoch making – beginning an era of health based on natural living.

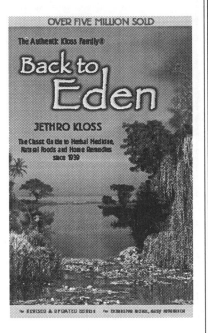

OVER FIVE MILLION SOLD

The Authentic Kloss Family®

Back to Eden

JETHRO KLOSS

The Classic Guide to Herbal Medicine, Natural Foods and Home Remedies since 1939

~ REVISED & UPDATED EDITION ~ EXTENSIVE INDEX, EASY REFERENCE

Trade Paper	ISBN 0-940985-09-8	936p	$14.95
Hardcover	ISBN 0-940985-13-6	936p	$21.95
Mass Market	ISBN 0-940985-10-1	936p	$ 9.95

Available at bookstores and natural food stores nationwide, or order your copy directly by sending the appropriate amount for the binding of your choice plus $2.50 shipping/handling ($.75 s/h for each additional copy ordered at the same time) to:

Lotus Press, P O Box 325, Twin Lakes, WI 53181 USA
toll free order line: 800 824 6396   office phone: 262 889 8561
office fax: 262 889 8591   email: lotuspress@lotuspress.com
web site: www.lotuspress.com

Lotus Press is the publisher of a wide range of books and software in the field of alternative health, including Ayurveda, Chinese medicine, herbology, aromatherapy, Reiki and energetic healing modalities. Request our free book catalog.

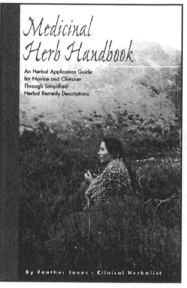

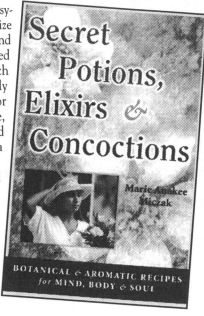